RISK MANAGEMENT FOR HOSPITALS

A Practical Approach

Bernard L. Brown, Jr., F.A.C.H.A.

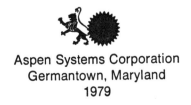

Aspen Systems Corporation
Germantown, Maryland
1979

Library of Congress Cataloging in Publication Data

Brown, Bernard L.
Risk management for hospitals: a practical approach.

Bibliography: p. 171
Includes index.
1. Hospitals—Administration.   2. Risk management.
3. Hospitals—Safety measures.   4. Tort liability
of hospitals—United States.   I. Title.
RA971.B86   658.1'53   78-31925
ISBN 0-89443-090-4

Library of Congress Catalog Card Number: 78-31925
ISBN: 0-89443-090-4

Printed in the United States of America

1 2 3 4 5

To my wife and my God
for their help and inspiration

Table of Contents

Forewords

This book on a timely subject, *risk management,* presents a practical approach to a very complex concern of the health care field. The loss of charitable immunity, coupled with an ever-increasing public expectation that the health care institution is not only a guarantor to cure the disease or injury which required its services but a warrantor of the results of its treatment as well, has placed the hospital in a unique, vulnerable position. Public expectations plus public dissatisfaction because of the rapid cost escalation that has occurred, particularly during the last decade, create an environment that requires hospitals to develop risk management programs in some form.

Even if the present-day environment were less litigious, the need to make certain that negative or untoward results are minimized would make this book a valuable addition to the hospital field. Patients do not become hospitalized to be injured, but cured.

The loss prevention or liability control processes presented in this study are based upon the management philosophy of an outstanding practicing chief executive officer of an excellently managed institution.

The relevance of the subject matter, its organization, and its presentation make this book understandable and informative.

W. Daniel Barker, FACHA
Administrator
The Crawford W. Long Memorial Hospital
of Emory University
Atlanta, Georgia
(Chairman, Board of Trustees,
American Hospital Association—1979)

I am grateful that Bernard L. Brown, Jr., a distinguished colleague, has taken the time to provide the practicing profession of hospital administration with a practical guide for organizing risk management programs. For several years the literature of our field has been heavy with articles by insurance specialists, attorneys, engineers, and others with specific expertise, who, while definitely making a contribution, have tended to give risk management an aura of mystery. If generalist chief executives have been at all mystified by the term "risk management," even though they well know they have managed while ever aware of risks, Mr. Brown's book easily clears the air and makes the subject appear familiar indeed.

Obviously, through statute, case law, regulations and accreditation standards, we are quite aware of our vulnerabilities in terms of a safe environment for both patients and employees as well as the quality of care. Often, however, safety programs, infection control activities, and quality assurance have been separate, uncoordinated efforts without central organization and thrust.

At my own hospital, we have only recently organized what we intend to be a comprehensive and effective risk management program, including the appropriate committees working with a full-time risk manager. This new book, by a seasoned hospital executive, could not be more timely as a guide distilled from actual experience. I look upon this volume as a fortunate resource, and commend it to every hospital executive who is beginning or reorganizing his approaches to loss prevention or liability controls. To those who have not yet established centrally coordinated risk management programs, I would urge such hospital managements to seriously consider doing so.

Author Brown reminds us that this is more than a safety program, as we commonly know it, though certainly building and fire safety are encompassed in risk management. Rather, it is identifying all potential areas for liability exposure, particularly including all aspects of patient care, and establishing programs and corrective measures that will improve patient care and reduce possibility of harm. Risk management in a hospital, as Mr. Brown points out, is anything but a negative program, for its chief objective is the elimination of problems that can result in harm to patients, employees, or the organization.

I agree; the time for comprehensive risk management programs is *now*. I also agree that participation of the medical staff is crucial for realizing the full objectives of such a program. But the important thing is . . . let's begin. This book tells administrators how to go about it in the management terms they understand.

Norman D. Burkett, FACHA
President
Hamilton Memorial Hospital
Dalton, Georgia
(Chairman, American College of
Hospital Administrators—1978)

Preface

Several years ago, our institution was faced with an unbelievably high professional liability (malpractice) insurance premium on the basic policy that we had carried for many years. This was the third consecutive year that this cost had risen 50 percent or more. After much analysis, preparation, and last-minute soul searching, we chose to follow the self-insurance route for professional and general liability in our hospital. At the time, this made us pioneers in our area of the country in regard to such a program.

Shortly afterwards, the Southeastern Regional Director of the American Hospital Association asked me to be a participant in a seminar to present our risk management program in a case study forum. I remember naively asking, "What is risk management?" This was the first time I ever heard the term risk management used in the context of hospital administration. He proceeded to inform me that you are supposed to have a risk management program if you have a self-insurance plan. At that point, I decided that I had better look into this new hospital term, *risk management*. Because of this interest and our hospital's implementation of a risk management program, I have subsequently been asked to participate in other state, regional, and national conferences on this subject.

The risk management program that currently exists in our hospital was used extensively as a resource for this book. The governing board of our institution is progressive in terms of activities that improve patient services but conservative in respect to the financial management of hospital funds. I mention this because the risk management program that will be described in this book was born in this type of environment. This fact alone leads me to the conclusion that risk management can be a *practical* solution to certain institutional problems.

This book is my first attempt at a composition of this magnitude, and it has proved to be a mammoth undertaking for someone who is primarily a practitioner and not much of a theorist. Its preparation was completed in nine months, primarily at night and on weekends, in an attempt to make this timely information available to hospitals and related organizations as expeditiously as possible. It will become quite clear to the reader that this venture into authorship did not result in a scholarly work of great literary value. However, it will hopefully serve as a helpful guide on a crucial subject to a very challenged industry.

Conscious effort has been made to present this material in a simple and concise manner. Layman's language is used primarily for two basic reasons: first, highly specialized jargon does not impart the desired practical understanding; second, my vocabulary is basically limited to everyday conversational words.

Although one cannot help but expound somewhat on philosophy, the purpose of this effort is to provide a *how to* approach to this new program, which is gaining increasing popularity. Numerous principles are suggested and many examples are cited in an attempt to remain as practical as possible in the presentation.

Finally, I strongly believe in the risk management approach to loss control and liability prevention in hospitals or I would not have made this effort. However, like the Sunday School teacher, the author may have gotten more out of this literary exercise than the reader. I personally have grown tremendously in my understanding of the subject matter presented herein. My only hope and prayer is that you who are interested will be enlightened and more knowledgeable of this new hospital administration program after reading this text.

Bernard L. Brown, Jr.
March 1979

Acknowledgments

In the course of preparing a manuscript such as this, many help and lend. support, either directly or indirectly. No doubt the person who contributed most was my secretary, Alta W. Shaw, who persevered through the many drafts and changes necessitated by an inexperienced author. Additionally, those who directly assisted include: Thompson A. Arrendale, Samuel D. Bishop, Glenn J. Black, Jr., John S. Bowling, Brue S. Chandler III, Betty C. Fricks, R. Warren Gordon, Elizabeth A. Hamilton, W. Ernie McCollum, Bonnie S. Phipps, J. P. VanLandingham, and Jane M. Wallace.

Others have significantly influenced the development of the many thoughts, ideas, and concepts that are presented herein, and in addition provided the moral support and encouragement that led to this presentation. I especially wish to name the following: W. Daniel Barker, Roy E. Barnes, Norman D. Burkett, James E. Ferguson, Frederick H. Gibbs, Leon I. Gintzig, Ph.D., Frank D. Holcomb, Matthew F. McNulty, Jr., Sc.D., members of The Cobb County Kennestone Hospital Authority, and—particularly—Reverend and Mrs. Bernard L. Brown, Sr.

Introduction

In an institution as complicated, diversified, and dynamic as a hospital, new programs and plans are almost constantly being introduced and considered. In this setting, it is not unusual for new activities to come into existence and overnight become a beneficial ongoing function within the organization. The emergence of many of these activities has resulted directly from technological and sociological advances in the health care field. Others, particularly those in the management realm, have been developed to fulfill specific needs that have arisen out of the organization's complex nature.

The administration of a hospital is probably more difficult and challenging than that of any other institution. For a hospital to progress in effectiveness and efficiency, maximum effort needs to be given to an objective of overcoming these administrative difficulties and challenges. Management programs with this objective should continuously be sought and given serious attention as part of the hospital's administrative effort. *Risk management* is one of these programs that deserve consideration.

The approach used in such consideration must be a *practical* one, for too often programs conceived as good theory result in poor practice. This has been particularly true in hospitals, where all sorts of pressures are brought to bear in regard to pet projects. Initially, risk management will probably be no one's pet (except possibly the hospital's governing body and administration who are faced with paying the high cost resulting from institutional liability). However, such a program could become everyone's pet if it results in limited resources being reallocated from institutional losses to personal gains.

Operational activities founded in industrial and business settings are more and more finding their way into health care institutions. The traditional philosophies of *quality at any price* and *let us alone because we are in the business of saving lives* are being abandoned in many hospitals. New rules are being promoted that support the premise that quality service can be provided at a more reasonable price. Quality assurance and risk management programs have been in existence in many industrial plants and other business enterprises for a number of years. The vulnerability of these organizations to liability losses may have promoted earlier interest in this area. Despite the motives behind the creation of such programs, these activities have become mainstays in many industries and businesses. It will be interesting to observe if risk management will be another example of organizational activity rooted in another industry that in time finds its place and proves its worth in health care institutions.

The main thrust of this presentation is toward those institutions that are giving consideration to the establishment of the risk management function within their organizations. Much of the material will also be useful to hospitals that already have an active program.

An evaluation of a hospital function such as risk management requires an understanding of that function's purpose, objectives, requirements, organization, and means. The following chapters attempt to impart this understanding from a practical standpoint. At the conclusion of each chapter is a checklist that reviews the chapter's content by asking pertinent questions about the subject matter. These checklists will hopefully assist in developing a better understanding of risk management as a hospital function.

Chapter 1

Perspective of Risk Management in Hospitals

Risk management is the term for a relatively new approach in the health care field. This approach encompasses many operational elements that have been in existence for a long time in the hospital setting. The development of a risk management program does not necessarily mean starting from scratch. It does, however, generally involve a change in emphasis, a reorganization, and better coordination of existing activities. An understanding of this point may help dispel the reluctance of many institutions to initiate this much needed approach.

DEFINITION OF RISK MANAGEMENT

On the surface, these words, "risk" and "management," seem to be somewhat paradoxical when placed together to describe a program. *Risk* has a negative connotation and implies the need for avoidance, while *management* is generally considered an active effort to achieve positive results. However, a program that provides positive avoidance of negative results is not paradoxical. It is instead part of a good overall management program.

Risk management in the organizational setting might as easily be called loss prevention or liability control. Its purpose is to eliminate problems that may result in harm to the organization, its staff, and, most important, its public.

Many definitions of risk management can be found in current literature. An examination of these definitions indicates many basic similarities. For example, risk management is defined as the science for the identification, evaluation, and treatment of the risk of financial loss.[1] The procedure for dealing with risk (i.e., risk management) can be defined as the science of detecting, evaluating, financing, and reducing risk of financial loss.[2] The purpose of a basic risk management program is to (1) avoid the causes of loss,

(2) lessen the operational and financial effects created by losses that are unavoidable, and (3) provide for inevitable losses at the lowest practical cost.[3] Risk management represents a functional planning approach to risk problems, particularly those of professional liability for hospitals. The process includes three steps: risk identification, risk control, and risk financing.[4] The purpose of a basic risk management program is to minimize the cost of loss from basic risk through identifying, measuring, and controlling these basic risks.[5]

There is often a tendency to look at new programs such as this only in terms of their financial appropriateness. Risk management in a health care institutional setting should primarily be considered a means of improving and maintaining quality patient care. The area of loss control should be viewed first from the humanitarian standpoint and second from the financial standpoint.[6]

THE EXTERNAL ENVIRONMENT

Hospital and health care costs in the United States have increased at such a phenomenal rate in recent years that the industry as a whole, as well as individual institutions, is under tremendous pressure to stop the upward spiral. The patient demands relief, the insurance carriers quote higher premiums, the news media editorialize reform, government threatens further intervention, the doctor develops a persecution complex, and the hospital laments, "What's an institution to do?" The general public asks, "Are we getting our money's worth and, even if we are, can we afford it?"

The once sacred hospital, the haven for the care of the sick and injured, the great institution that was immune from criticism because of its high charitable purpose, no longer wears a halo. The hospital, like many others with institutional establishment status, is coming under increasing scrutiny and is becoming more vulnerable to the hazards of the traditional business world.

It seems that the hospital as an institution is even suffering to some degree from the success it enjoyed during the past century. The modern hospital is a product of rapid technological and sociological advances. Today's happenings in the hospital environment would have been considered miracles 50 years ago. Physical and mental health care have made dramatic strides from art to science during this period.

These advances have been vividly demonstrated to the hospitals' public through the medium of television. Some of the most popular television programs in recent years have centered around hospitals and doctors. The "Marcus Welby"/"Medical Center"/"Emergency" images are often difficult ones for health care providers to live up to. In real life, cures are not as prevalent nor do those being "cured" always live happily ever after.

High expectations are in the minds of most patients when they enter the health care system. In reality the risk involved in institutional health care is secondary to them at the time of entry. A great degree of dissatisfaction is often the result of miracles unrealized, of problems left unsolved or only partially solved, or of the failure of the system to avoid the inevitable.

In addition, specialization now dominates the health care field. This has resulted in confusion not only among the recipients of health care but also among the various providers. In the eyes of the hospitals' public, overspecialization is analogous to the depersonalization of human beings.[7]

Our changing society has put the hospital in a unique position with respect to today's emphasis on consumerism, individual rights, fiduciary responsibilities, public disclosure, and conflict of interest. The hospital has difficulty in defining its role in this complicated system. This results in difficulties in the hospital's adapting itself to societal pressures.

In examining roles within the health care system, an interesting array of characters is identified. Professionals, paraprofessionals, nonprofessionals, specialists, generalists, highly skilled, semiskilled, nonskilled, highly educated, poorly educated, rich, poor, upper class, middle class, lower class, capitalists, socialists—on and on go the descriptions of people found in the hospital setting.

The hospital's *customers* are doctors. In general, they are the only ones who can order services from the institution. Doctors decide what patients are to be admitted and when, they decide which services are to be provided, and they decide when and under what circumstances patients leave the hospital. However, doctors, as customers, do not consume any of the services generated by the hospital; the hospital's *consumers* are its patients. The health care institution is unusual in this respect; its customer is different from its consumer. This phenomenon creates the need for a tremendous amount of good communication and understanding on the part of the parties involved in this relationship. The complexities created by this situation can result in confusion and misunderstanding that can, in turn, lead to serious problems.

In general, external attitudes toward the hospital are changing. The awe of the institution is fading; accountability is becoming a requirement. The individual who uses the hospital and the public that provides support are demanding explanations of the hospital's role in society.

INTERNAL ATTITUDES

In the early stages of development of the modern hospital, typical hospital workers often considered themselves similar to missionaries. They worked for salaries or wages far below those received by persons with comparable training and experience in other fields. Hospital workers performed tasks that, in some cases, bordered on being hazardous and that, in general, were undesirable, overly demanding, and unappreciated. Because of the common bond of work directed toward a noble purpose, a family atmosphere among workers was prevalent in the health care institutional setting.

This atmosphere seems to be changing with the increasing sophistication of the health care delivery system and concomitant technological advances associated with a large degree of ultraspecialization and improved methods of financing. During these developments, the hospital began to take its rightful place as one of the most necessary and most important community institutions. Likewise, the hospital workers' status grew, and high self-esteem and expectations followed. As images changed, hospital workers were torn between their heritage of service and personal sacrifice and their new expectations of increased financial rewards and community status. Unionization of hospital workers became more prevalent in some areas of the country as attitudes changed.

Hospitals, like other established institutions providing "human" services, began to receive complaints of loss of identity and individuality of those served, lack of the personal touch by those serving, and general deterioration of services. Some of the older workers began commenting, "When we were few in number and like a family, people cared about each other. The boss cared about us, and we cared about our patients."

It seems that some problems of *organizational* family life are parallel to those of *personal* family life in today's complex society. The problems of alienation, separation, division, liberation, and generation gaps have become common in both of these areas of the total life experience. When institution and individual, labor and management, supervisor and worker, and working peers come together within the organization, many of the same problems surface as do in a family. Husbands and wives, parents and children, brothers and sisters have these problems. Many of the emotions that create these problems in both homes and institutions are identical. Such emotions as jealousy, envy, pride, greed, and fear seem to provide the underlying roots.

One of the basic problems with society today, according to many psychology and sociology experts, is the deterioration of the family. Some have tied escalating delinquency and crime rates, growth in poverty levels, poor mental and physical health, and many other types of adverse conditions to the decline in well-being of the home and family. When people consider the organizations in which they work as their vocational homes, they can easily identify many of the same problems and pressures that are present in their personal homes.

The hospital, being a labor intense work place, suffers from inherent *people* problems. Relatively high turnover rates, poor morale, personality conflicts, and other personnel-related problems are often common challenges that face administrators in hospitals.

Another complexity in the hospital organizational structure is the institution's previously noted relationship with physicians. Doctors seem to be neither fish nor fowl in terms of this relationship. The hospital can be held liable for certain acts of physicians, even though it exercises limited control over physicians' activities within the institution. However, there seems to be a fine line between controlling the practice of medicine, that only physicians are licensed to perform, and infringing upon it. Therefore, a somewhat gray area exists, and each situation must be viewed individually when an attempt is made to define responsibility and authority that affect the hospital's exposure to risk.

In general, the internal atmosphere in the modern hospital is complicated by the dynamics of the organization and by the complexity of the relationships that exist there.

LIABILITY INSURANCE TRENDS

A recognized crisis exists in malpractice and professional liability in the health care field. Not only has the cost of insurance risen to astronomical levels but, in some cases, liability insurance has become unavailable.

In one hospital, for example, over a 15-year period the rates of a basic liability insurance program provided by a commercial insurance carrier rose from 2 cents per dollar to 50 cents per dollar for comparable coverage. This increase occurred despite the fact that this particular hospital had experienced less than average claims and settlements. Another hospital's malpractice insurance has risen from $.79 per patient day in 1974 to $11.20 per patient day in 1977, or almost five percent of the total cost of caring for the patient.[8] These types of experiences are cited over and over in conversations among hospital administrators.

Insurance companies give many reasons for this tremendous growth in liability insurance cost. Some of these include the astronomical judgments and awards by the courts in recent years, the general trend to sue at the drop of a hat in our society in general, the removal of charitable and government immunity from many hospitals, actuarial projections that are attuned to spiraling inflation and escalating cost of living, and more lawyers needing to earn a living. The list could go on and on.

Whatever the reasons, there is no doubt that a problem exists. In response to the problem hospitals began to seek out alternatives to the conventional commercial liability insurance programs. Such programs as self-insurance plans, captive and shared insurance programs, and "going bare" have become in vogue, with differing degrees of success. Because of the acuteness of some situations, legislation has been passed in several states to deal with some of the problems related to the availability and cost of malpractice insurance.

Of equal importance to the need for finding a means to provide an adequate liability insurance program is the need to seek out ways to reduce some of the causes of this crisis. Ultimately, this should help to control losses that result from these causes.

THE MANAGEMENT PROCESSES

Management, of course, is pertinent because loss prevention or liability control is a *management* program; specifically, a *risk management* program. According to most philosophers on the subject, management is a set of processes. These processes are defined in various ways, but all of these definitions generally boil down to the activities that must be successfully performed to insure the result for which management exists. The format of these processes or activities is usually the creation of the individual manager. In other words, most definitions agree that management processes exist but that specific processes differ among individuals.

The processes of management that this author attempts to follow include:

- *Planning*—Establishing obtainable goals and the means of accomplishing them.
- *Organizing*—Developing and staffing an organizational structure and system designed to obtain these goals.
- *Directing*—Providing leadership to the organization.
- *Coordinating*—Promoting understanding among all organization components through communication and education.
- *Monitoring*—Exercising follow-up and control procedures to insure progress toward objectives.

In managing any enterprise conscientious effort to follow defined processes is essential. By applying the above management processes to risk reduction or loss control, the framework is laid for creating and operating a good risk management program. First, *plan* the program with specific objectives aimed at eliminating risk. Second, *organize* a structure and system with appropriate staff support necessary for the program to operate successfully. Third, provide *direction* through adequate commitment, support, and emphasis at all organizational levels. Fourth, keep the organization informed and involved through *coordination* of activities. Finally, constantly *monitor* the effectiveness of the program so that it can adapt to the needs of the organization and accomplish its purpose.

CONCLUSION

Risk management seems unlike most other programs found in hospitals. The name of this program may seem to imply a hard, mechanistic, impersonal process. But risk management is only a term for a very serious subject. It sounds like a business term, drawn from the realm of pure financial management with minimal human involvement. Placed in a hospital setting, though, the reverse is true. Here, risk management is dominated by the human element.[9]

A program such as risk management needs to be perceived in the context of today's hospital environment. Probably ten or even five years ago, a decision to implement such a program would have been automatically discounted. However, because of the many pressures and challenges currently associated with institutional liability, many hospitals are beginning seriously to consider inclusion of risk management programs.

PERSPECTIVE OF RISK MANAGEMENT CHECKLIST

___ Is a risk management program being considered in your hospital?

___ Does a basic understanding of the definition of risk management and its purpose exist?

___ Is the external environment surrounding your hospital changing relative to increased risk potential?

___ Are the attitudes of those within your organization becoming more impersonal resulting in deterioration of hospital services?

___ Is the availability of liability insurance decreasing and / or is the cost increasing dramatically?

___ Are a set of management processes used in your hospital and can they be applied to a risk management program?

Note: This checklist is not meant to be all inclusive, nor does it require absolute adherence. Its purpose is to stimulate thought and redirect attitudes toward the establishment of a risk management program.

NOTES

1. T. Dankmyer and J. Groves, "Taking Steps for Safety's Sake," *Hospitals, JAHA,* May 16, 1977, p. 60.

2. J. Ashby, S. Stephens, and S. Pearson, "Elements in Successful Risk Reduction Programs," *Hospital Progress,* July 1977, p. 60.

3. J. O'Connell, "Risk Management for Hospitals," *Hospital Progress,* November 1974, p. 40.

4. M. Thistle, "A Look at the Causes and Possible Solutions," *Risk Management,* July 1977, p. 10.

5. A. Clark, "Management Approaches to Basic Risks," *Hospital Progress,* November 1974, p. 43.

6. "FAH Manual Outlines Control Programs on Risk Management for Hospital Use," *FAH Review,* February 1977, p. 13.

7. Thistle, p. 10.

8. "The Decline and Demise of the Community Hospital," *Insights* (Northfield, Ill. : J. Lloyd Johnson Associates, 1978), p. 5.

9. M. Grayson, "Risk Management: New Focus for Traditional Functions," *The Hospital Medical Staff,* May 1978, p. 12.

Chapter 2

Prerequisites for a Risk Management Program

Development of a risk management program does not necessarily mean starting from scratch, although it generally involves a change of emphasis, reorganization, and better coordination of existing activities. Therefore, the logical place to start when considering such a program is with an inventory of existing activities. Where necessary the risk management philosophy must be applied to these existing functional elements. When reviewing organizational activities from a risk management perspective, most will fall within five basic categories: preventive, corrective, documentary, educational, and administrative.

The process of defining prerequisites for an effective risk management program is, in itself, a healthy organizational exercise that quickly will identify many of the weaknesses and needs that should be addressed while formalizing the institution's risk management program.

PREVENTIVE ACTIVITIES

One of the principal roles of any health care institution is to provide *quality* service. Quality in this context includes both the technical and the *personal* components of service rendered. All will agree that service must be technically proficient, but because health care is primarily a human service, it must be delivered in a personal, empathetic manner. Not only must the hospital's patients receive excellent service but they must also *believe* that quality care is being given. Any program or activity within the hospital that fosters personal as well as technical quality care can be classified as preventive in terms of the risk management program.

The American Hospital Association has taken a strong stand relative to risk prevention in hospitals. The AHA believes that the key solution to malpractice problems is the implementation of programs of prevention that will reduce risk to patients.[1]

Patient Relations

The relationships that patients have with organizational representatives are the most important ones that exist in the hospital setting. However, in some cases, these interpersonal relationships are neglected, become secondary, and are taken for granted.

Initially, one must recognize that a hospital is a service organization; its product is patient services. The nature of a service organization is different from that of most product-oriented industrial or business ventures. It also can be argued that a hospital is different from most other types of service organizations. The main distinguishing characteristic is that the hospital provides services that consumers would rather do without. If institutionalized patients were asked, "Would you rather be somewhere else today than here at the hospital?" their answers would support this premise. This characteristic poses a difficult problem for institutional staffs charged with the responsibility of providing these undesired services. It takes unique, specially motivated individuals to accept the responsibility required in a health care institutional setting. A sincere acknowledgment of this responsibility by the institution and its staff is the first step in developing a good patient relations program.

Ombudsmen Programs

In recent years some hospitals have incorporated formal patient representative programs within their organizational structures in an attempt to personalize services. What is needed, according to T. Chittenden, is the best attempt possible to communicate with the patient.[2] We do not think well of attempts to substitute a rote recitation for genuine communication.[3]

These programs generally assign representatives to patients to assist in fulfilling patients' personal needs and solving their individual problems. The acceptance of these and other ombudsmen programs has been excellent, but their financial feasibility and appropriateness may be questioned in these days when great emphasis is placed on cost containment. In most organizations the patient-relations function is primarily delegated to those front-line employees involved in direct patient contact.

As an alternative, some institutions have developed less sophisticated programs, such as the use of telephone answering services that are available 24 hours a day. However, such hot-line programs require immediate follow-up to inquiries and problems if patients and their families are to have confidence in this means of expressing their needs and desires. The patient advocate concept in various forms is gaining increased support as an important tool in improving the quality of care, thereby reducing claims against hospitals.[4]

Other Programs

Recent trends in patient care seem to be back to the basics. Primary nursing care and the use of the nursing process have again become popular in many health care institutions.[5] In theory, such concepts bring the nurse back to the bedside and assist in developing a personal relationship between nurse and patient.

Hospitals have begun to realize the need to involve family members in the total health care activities of the patient. Family support from both a physical and a mental standpoint is part of the overall treatment plan. Conveniences and activities to assist in making families more comfortable and more a part of the overall therapy program are becoming a part of many institutions. These techniques are being used to reduce apprehension experienced both by patients and by their families.

Satisfying the spiritual needs of patients is becoming universally recognized as part of their total health care. The use of trained hospital chaplains and counselors as well as volunteer ministers from the community has become an integral phase in the patient care process in most hospitals.

It is important that patients have both formal and informal means of expressing their opinions and evaluating the services given them during their stay in the hospital. Patient service questionnaire programs are very helpful in this regard (Exhibit 2-1). It is important that the information gathered from such efforts not be misused but be thoroughly evaluated to identify problems, strengths, and weaknesses in areas where improvement is needed. This information should be used throughout the entire organization, up to and including the highest policy-making level within the institution. The governing body of the organization needs to have an accurate feel for the status of the institution's relations with its patients on a continuing basis. There is no question that a good patient-relations program in any hospital is one of the most effective risk-prevention activities available.

Public Relations

Most large hospitals have full-time public or community relations directors or staffs to manage ongoing programs. Even in the smallest hospitals, the same needs, challenges, and problems exist. Therefore, such activities should be assigned as a responsibility of some individual on the staff, even if it is only on a part-time basis. The administrator, assistant administrator, or an appropriate department head or supervisor may well assume this function

Exhibit 2-1 Patient Service Questionnaire

(Hospital Slogan)

The care and comfort of our patients is our chief concern. To accomplish this end, we are constantly striving to improve the service we render. It is only through constructive evaluation and criticism that we can improve. In this regard, we would like for you to answer the questions listed below. Please feel free to express your opinions frankly, and return to us. Thank you for your assistance and cooperation.

(Name and Signature)

	Excellent	Good	Average	Poor
1. General impression of hospital	___	___	___	___
2. Treatment by personnel in:				
Admitting Office				
Laboratory	___	___	___	___
Radiology (X-Ray)	___	___	___	___
Electroencephalography (EEG)	___	___	___	___
Cardiology (EKG)	___	___	___	___
Respiratory Therapy	___	___	___	___
Rehabilitation Medicine	___	___	___	___
Emergency Services	___	___	___	___
Labor and Delivery Rooms	___	___	___	___
Surgical Suite	___	___	___	___
3. Nursing Service:				
Day Shift, 7 a.m. to 3 p.m.				
Evening Shift, 3 p.m. to 11 p.m.	___	___	___	___
Night Shift, 11 p.m. to 7 a.m.	___	___	___	___
4. Food you were served:				
Regular diet				
Special diet	___	___	___	___
5. Room you were assigned:				
Housekeeping services				
Laundry and linen	___	___	___	___
Maintenance services	___	___	___	___
6. Treatment of your visitors	___	___	___	___
7. Financial arrangements handled by our business office	___	___	___	___

IMPORTANT: Were all questions answered and problems either solved or explained satisfactorily when presented to any hospital representative?   YES ____   NO ____

COMMENTS AND SUGGESTIONS FOR IMPROVEMENT: _____

_____

Miss, Mrs., Mr. _____ Room _____ Date _____
              (Welcomed but not necessary)
Address _____ Zip _____

Source: Adaptation of form used by Kennestone Hospital, Marietta, Georgia, 1978.

effectively. The use of consultant services has also proved effective relative to public relations programs.

The News Media

Among the most important functions of the public relations program is news media relations. The hospital's image within the community setting is partly dependent on its projection through the various media forms. A hospital portrayed in a negative manner tends to be more susceptible to liability hazards, whereas one projected positively seems to be less litigation prone. However, it should be made clear that the public cannot be fooled for long in this regard. A good image of a bad service will not endure, but a bad image of a good service within a community can prevail if institutional and personal relationships are poor.

There seem to be two basic approaches to media relations. The first is promotional or educational; the second is a reactionary approach. It is always more desirable to anticipate a need for public education or institutional promotion and then to act in an effort to fill the need before it becomes apparent. Of course, at times the institution will be faced with the need to react publicly to problems or negative situations that have already occurred. When this happens, an honest yet discreet manner should be used in facing such issues. The highest ethical conduct is also imperative in these instances.

The Community

When discussing relationships between the hospital and its community, a key word is integration. The hospital must integrate its operation with community interests, involvement, and participation. Likewise, members of the hospital staff must integrate themselves into the activities of the community.

Generally, involvement at the governing level of the hospital by representatives of the general public and community is very helpful and healthy. If the organizational or corporate structure does not provide for this representation, advisory committee input should be developed.

Many hospitals encourage and support, morally and/or financially, staff member participation in local community and church activities. This is not only healthy for the individual's overall personal development but it also provides great advantages in strengthening relationships between community and hospital.

Possibly the strongest and most effective community relations programs that exist in hospitals are their volunteer programs. Volunteers provide augmentary and supportive services. In addition they prove to be an excellent means of relating the institution to the community. Volunteers in hospitals today include all types, ages, and both sexes from many walks of life. The largest volunteer force is usually the auxiliary or volunteer service organization. In many institutions, particularly public and governmental, the hospital governing body members are volunteers, and they generally serve without any remuneration. Some hospitals have volunteer chaplaincy programs made up of local clergymen. A tremendous potential for good community relations exists among these resources.

Personnel Relations

Effective personnel programs are essential ingredients of overall opera-, tional effectiveness. The cost of labor in a hospital is second to no other single expense. Therefore, activities geared to obtaining high productivity while maintaining a caring attitude on the part of the employees are certainly preventive in terms of risk management. Some of the basic functions of a personnel program include:

- wage and salary administration
- fringe benefits
- position control and job classification
- employee recruitment, orientation, training, and education
- employee evaluation
- employee grievance procedures
- employee conduct procedures
- personnel/employment analyses and reporting systems
- other related activities

Good personnel relations programs improve patient services and increase the potential for reducing risk and controlling loss in hospitals. Perhaps specific examples of the effectiveness of such programs will be helpful at this point. This author, in collaboration with Linda McFarland, director of educational services at Kennestone Hospital (Marietta, Ga.), prepared an article on the improvement of patient services through good employee relations programs, from which the following ideas are taken:[6]

Good employee morale and esprit de corps among the work force, which ultimately lead to good patient services, are often mentioned in the same breath with higher salaries and greater fringe benefits. Certainly these incentives are important, but they are not the only nor necessarily the most significant factors in recruiting and retaining excellent employees. Such employees are the main ingredient needed to provide excellent patient services in a hospital.

The hospital family has a significant impact on the attitude, motivation, and effectiveness of an employee, just as an individual's personal family environment greatly influences his or her personal life. Therefore, those programs that encourage a healthy organizational family atmosphere in a hospital ultimately improve patient care.

Several programs directed at creating an atmosphere of participation and involvement both in the operation and in the philosophy of the organization have proved successful at Kennestone Hospital.

A Hospital Slogan

The initial step in an attempt to form an employee relations program directed toward patient-centered services, was a contest among employees to create a slogan for Kennestone. Members of the Personnel Committee of the hospital's governing board served as judges. Hospital policy guidelines, including Kennestone's own patient "bill of rights," were used by employees to develop the more than 200 entries that were submitted. Finalists were selected, and the winner was announced at the hospital's annual employee recognition banquet. The winning slogan was "Professionally We Serve, Personally We Care." This phrase now appears on most official documents that originate in the hospital. More important it has become a philosophical attitude that has been integrated into Kennestone's administration and operation.

Interestingly, answers on the hospital's patient service questionnaires showed that ratings from patients improved significantly after the slogan was placed into use. This improvement has been maintained. During the past several years, Kennestone's facilities have grown significantly in size and scope. Such growth often results in depersonalization and a general deterioration in caring. However, the slogan has served as a reminder of Kennestone's purpose and philosophy during this period of change.

Administration Personnel Exchange

Good communications is one key to an effective organization, and it certainly fosters good organizational family relationships. A program to improve communications, the Administration Personnel Exchange (APE), was initiated to provide a mechanism for direct communication between Kennestone's top administrative officials and the front-line workers. The administration uses this program to help bridge the management/labor gap during a time of dynamic change in the health care field and to provide information to improve the hospital's operation. Excerpts from the initial announcement of this program follow.

It has become mod to refer to a new program by its initials. A new program which we are starting turned out to have an unusual set of initials, APE, which stands for Administration Personnel Exchange. The philosophy of this program is as follows:

- It is easy for a chief executive to become isolated from the organization. There are many organization levels between the administrator and the front-line workers who are getting the job done. An administrator does not have the opportunity to get to know personnel on an individual basis in an organization as large as ours. Even if possible, it could be detrimental to the organization for the administrator to develop informal relationships with employees for this could usurp the authority of the middle levels of management and supervision and reduce their effectiveness.
- In an attempt to get to know hospital employees better (their problems, their frustrations, their objectives, their motivations, and so forth) and, at the same time, support the formal organizational structure, the APE program will be initiated on a trial basis. Its purpose is to create an exchange of ideas between hospital personnel and the administrator.
- Fifteen to eighteen employees each month will be selected at random by the payroll computer. They will be invited to attend the one hour APE session and notified a week in advance to give them time to organize thoughts and formulate questions. Following the meeting, each is free and encouraged to share information obtained with fellow employees.

The first session and subsequent meetings uncovered many inconsistencies in the interpretation and practice of hospital policies and procedures. The sessions prompted action by the administration to change policies and procedures in certain cases, to enforce some that were not previously emphasized, and to eliminate others that were meaningless or unnecessary. The program enabled top administration of the hospital better to understand the everyday problems and frustrations of the hospital employee. It also enabled employees at the grassroots level to gain a better understanding, and, to a degree, greater participation in the management of the hospital.

The administrator must be careful not to make improper commitments when approached about certain subjects during a session. A conscious effort to support and not undermine the formal organization must be made.

Information obtained from employees was discussed in general terms with division and department heads after each session. It is important that the administrator does not violate the confidence of employees who have been open and direct in their discussion.

The program was well received. It proved more successful than originally anticipated and has produced many excellent byproducts. A change that has already occurred is an expansion of the program to include assistant administrator participation in APE sessions.

Employee Recognition

A positive approach to employee relations is far more effective than a negative one. A deserved pat on the back and an expression of appreciation for a job well done can prove to be valuable motivators toward good patient services. Formalizing employee recognition programs is usually necessary to insure consistency and continuity.

Some of the programs that have proved effective at Kennestone Hospital include:

- Employee of the Month. Nominations from hospital departments are screened and an outstanding employee is selected monthly. In addition to rewards (plaque, savings bond, and special parking space) for this selection, recognition is given in the hospital's monthly newsletter. The 12 monthly winners are candidates for Employee of the Year award.
- Annual Employee Recognition Dinner. Employees with extended service are honored, and the Employee of the Year is announced.
- Wall of Honor. Portraits of employees with 25-year tenure are displayed in a lobby area to acknowledge their service to the institution.
- Kindness Cards. Thank-you notes are sent to employees when their names are specifically mentioned in letters or questionnaires from patients. Records of these expressions of appreciation are kept in personnel files (Exhibit 2-2).
- Christmas turkeys and small birthday gifts are presented to all employees annually.
- Contests in such areas as safety, nonsmoking, and weight watching are held periodically. Other recognition activities are also implemented from time to time.

Such activities create an atmosphere of participation and involvement not only in the operation but also in the philosophy of an institution. Employees who feel that they are truly important and contributing members of a hospital team will seek to provide good service. This employee attitude serves as a useful tool within a risk management program.

Medical Staff Relations

The physician/hospital relationship comes close to being one of the most complex relationships—possibly unique—in any modern organizational structure.

Exhibit 2-2 Kindness Card

---

*A Compliment For*_____

From _____

Patient's (or family) Name

(Hospital Logo)

Thank you for making another friend for our hospital!

F

(Hospital)

A patient specifically mentioned your name in compliment-ing the hospital recently, so you are to be commended for promoting the high reputation of our hospital.

Because of you, we are living up to the high ideals of our purpose.

(Hospital Slogan)

B

Source: Adaptation of form used by Kennestone Hospital, Marietta, Georgia, 1978.

There often seems to be an inherent difference of philosophy between administrators and physicians relative to methods of reaching hospital objectives. This can possibly be attributed to the fact that the hospital administrator is trained as an *organization person* and the physician is educated primarily as an *individual.*

This difference has caused operational problems and often has resulted in many inefficiencies in the health care system. To resolve this dilemma, the administrator must recognize the individuality of physicians regarding treatment given their patients. The pattern of modern medicine practiced in the United States, which recognizes each patient as an individual, has resulted in a much higher level of care in comparison to that given when patient individuality is not recognized.

Concurrently, physicians must realize the need for organization and discipline to insure the best service for the greatest number of patients. One might compare the relationship of the physician and the hospital (or the hospital administrator) to that of the partners in an incompatible marriage. Listed below are nine factors that may contribute to this incompatibility.

The Incompatible Marriage[7]
Physician–Hospital

He (Physician)	She (Hospital)
1. He is a capitalist.	1. She practices a form of socialism.
2. He is a specialist.	2. She is multidisciplined.
3. He must control.	3. She cannot be controlled by one.
4. He resists regimentation.	4. She must have rules to survive.
5. He is oriented to one.	5. She must serve many concurrently.
6. He must make his own decisions.	6. Her decisions are determined by policy.
7. He is a conservative.	7. She is a liberal.
8. He is an idealist.	8. She is a realist.
9. He is an individualist.	9. She is an organization.

From the hospital's viewpoint, there are many methods and techniques that can be used to reduce the problems of incompatibility and improve the relationship between hospital and medical staff. Techniques for reducing conflict vary among institutions, depending on each organizational setup, and some have proved very effective.

Physician Involvement

Over the past several decades, the pros and cons of medical staff membership on hospital boards have been debated. Most professional organizations, particularly at the national level, have endorsed the concept of physician representation on hospital governing boards. This inclusion enhances communication between the medical staff and the governing body, and it allows input from the physician's viewpoint. When the medical staff feels that its viewpoint has been fairly represented in policy establishment, it will be quicker to accept hospital programs.

Other forms of communication between the hospital's governing board and the medical staff are also healthy. Joint meetings may be held in many different formats and settings. These tend to foster good communication and encourage mutual understanding, enabling further progress toward the common goal of providing excellent services.

While it is important that the medical staff viewpoint be integrated into hospital board activities, it is equally important that the hospital's governing body be provided means for constantly monitoring and reviewing the programs, progress, and problems of the staff. Individuals who make up hospital boards must be committed to the task of efficiently governing the facility. To accomplish this, they must be informed and committed to broadening their knowledge to keep pace with the fast-moving, technically oriented business of running a hospital. They are often lay people, in the sense of the technicalities of the hospital business; therefore, they should demand adequate explanation from all who are offering information, problems, and ideas for their consideration. This requirement will insure proper communication, which will result in better decisions made at the board level.

Many hospitals have learned that an excellent way to improve cooperation with the medical staff is to provide that staff with administrative support. Providing clerical help, not only in the area of medical information but also in the operational activities of the staff in general, has proved to be most effective in improving the function of the medical staff organization. Some large hospitals include a director of medical affairs as a part of the organizational structure to help insure effective medical staff activities. Many institutions without physicians on their administrative staffs have chosen to establish medical staff offices with secretarial support to assist elected staff officers in fulfilling their responsibilities.

A medical staff newsletter published by the hospital has become a popular means of keeping medical staff members informed and of communicating news, policies, procedures, and service activities. This may easily be a part of the regular hospital newsletter, a supplement to it, or a separate document designed specifically for this purpose.

Physician Opinions

Some institutions are using a technique called a medical staff opinion poll. This poll serves as an objective, thorough way to evaluate hospital services from the physician's viewpoint on a periodic basis (Exhibit 2–3).[8] This type of poll is most effective when maximum participation is obtained, the information is accurately tabulated, and true results are reported to all involved in the process, including medical staff members, department heads, and the governing body.

As cited above, the administrative/medical staff relationship can become strained and be the source of conflicts because of some of the inherent characteristics of this relationship. Therefore, it is important that the medical staff representatives be integrated into activities of the hospital, both at the governing, and at the administrative levels. It is also desirable that administrative input be developed within the medical staff organization. This is best accomplished by including appropriate members of the hospital's administrative team on medical staff committees.

There is no doubt that the relationship that exists between the hospital's medical staff and other members of the organization affects either positively or negatively the overall activities of the institution. Good, open, and constructive communication and an active liaison with the medical staff and its members are the best ways to insure a functional and effective hospital setting that fosters quality service.

Physical Environment

Providing a physical environment conducive to quality patient care as well as a setting that is as free as possible from risk and danger has been given great emphasis in recent years by the Joint Commission on the Accreditation of Hospitals (JCAH), state licensure agencies, and, particularly at the federal level, by OSHA and other mandated programs. The old motto of *safety first* when referring to facilities is popular again, and life safety code manuals are on the shelves of hospital administrators and engineers.

Every hospital should provide necessary emphasis and support to its environmental services not only because of regulations, standards, and laws, but also because they are essential elements of good patient care. Recent years have seen the elevation of these services to higher levels within the hospital organizational structure. It is common today to see assistant administrators or division heads with specific expertise in this area on the organization chart. In many hospitals, environmental services include not only the departments that clean and maintain the physical plant but also

Exhibit 2-3 Medical Staff Opinion Poll

Specialty: _____   Staff Membership: ☐ Active ☐ Associate ☐ Courtesy   Duration: _____ yrs.____

NURSING DEPARTMENTS	Supervision				Quality & Accuracy of Service				Promptness of Service				Patient Attitude Toward Service				Cooperation of Personnel			
	*E	G	F	P	E	G	F	P	E	G	F	P	E	G	F	P	E	G	F	P
Intensive Care Unit																				
Coronary Care Unit																				
Progressive CCU																				
Mental Health																				
Rehab Nsg.																				
4 South—Surgical																				
4 North—Surgical																				
5 South—Thoracic																				
5 North—Neuro																				
5 West—Ortho																				
6 West—Pediatrics																				
4 West—Medical																				
6 North—Medical																				
6 South—Oncology																				
GYN																				
Obstetrics																				
Labor & Delivery																				
Nursery																				
Clinic																				
Enterostomal Therapy																				
I.V. Therapy Team																				

SERVICES

- Emergency Services
- Surgical Suite & Recovery
- Laboratory
- Radiology
- Diagnostic Imaging
- Oncology Center
- Rehab Medicine
- Respiratory Therapy
- EKG
- EEG
- Utilization Review
- Pharmacy
- CSS
- Food Services
- Housekeeping
- Medical Records
- Admissions
- Social Services

- Emergency Services
- Surgical Suite & Recovery
- Laboratory
- Radiology
- Diagnostic Imaging
- Oncology Center
- Rehab Medicine
- Respiratory Therapy
- EKG
- EEG
- Utilization Review
- Pharmacy
- CSS
- Food Services
- Housekeeping
- Medical Records
- Admissions
- Social Services

ADMIN

Is the hospital's administration   ☐ pro   ☐ neutral toward   ☐ anti   Medical Staff?

Is it patient oriented?   ☐ yes   ☐ no

Is it cost conscious?   ☐ yes   ☐ no

Rating of administration   ☐ poor   ☐ average   ☐ good   ☐ excellent

{ OVERALL OPERATION IN COMPARISON TO PREVIOUS YEAR }
☐ HAS IMPROVED   ☐ REMAINED THE SAME   ☐ HAS DETERIORATED___

{ COMMENTS _____ }

(Use Back If Necessary)

*E (Excellent), G (Good), F (Fair), P (Poor)

Source: Adaptation of form used by Kennestone Hospital, Marietta, Georgia, 1978

23

those that provide supplies and materials used in the personal care of the patients.

While the hospital is required to provide physical surroundings conducive to excellent patient care, it is also under increasing economic pressure in this area because of the rapidly escalating cost of energy and utilities to support the physical plant. This dilemma—coupled with the booming technology of the health care industry that has resulted in ever-increasing expenses for supplies, materials, and equipment—poses unprecedented challenges to the environmental service departments. For these reasons, it is imperative that the hospital recognize the need to provide quality leadership for activities relating to the physical environment within it.

Maintenance Programs

Preventive maintenance programs developed and organized in a practical manner are most effective in avoiding unnecessary breakdowns in equipment and interruptions in services. However, it is necessary in such programs to insure that the effort and time involved produce effective results. A misconceived and misdirected preventive maintenance program both wastes time and is counterproductive.

The hospital environment includes not only the interior facilities but also the exterior properties and grounds. A good groundskeeping program not only enhances the hospital's appearance but also seeks to remove potential risks and hazards for those entering and leaving.

Quality control activities are a part of any good environmental services program. The monitoring of the facility itself, as well as the equipment and services provided within the hospital, is an essential function. In addition to basic maintenance and sanitation engineers and technicians, many hospitals today include medical equipment mechanics and biomedical engineers as part of the environmental service team. This assures appropriate monitoring and surveillance of environmental service programs. In many cases this team has assisted in reducing maintenance contract costs on highly technical equipment and services.

Zoning organization activities among environmental services is another approach being used by many hospitals. Mechanics and sanitation workers are assigned to specific areas within the hospital facility and given well-defined responsibility for environmental activities within those areas. This has proved an excellent means to insure proper care of often neglected engineering and sanitation functions. Other activities, including project planning and coordination, program review, educational and training activities, utility and basic service management, special services, and basic building maintenance, are also a part of most good environmental service functions.

Proper management of the hospital physical plant through effective environmental services is an essential ingredient when identifying risk-preventive activities of the institution.

Safety and Security

In recent years, many hospitals have followed the lead of other industries and established formal safety and security programs. Such programs are often headed by individuals with training, experience, and expertise in the areas of law enforcement and/or public safety. The hospital police force has come into existence during this period and has effectively filled the need for safety and security services that has increased in recent years.

The hospital seems, as never before, to be a target for crime and a place where violence can erupt. This possibly can be attributed to general trends within society as a whole. Drugs, food, and expensive supplies and equipment, which are attractive and easily sold on black markets, are used continuously as part of the hospital's everyday function. Mentally and emotionally disturbed patients and families are continuously present, bringing with them such potential problems as disruption in emergency wards and nursing units. The high concentration of female employees and workers attracts sexual offenders. Large parking lots around hospitals are filled with automobiles with hubcaps, batteries, and radios that are tempting to petty thieves. The amount of cash flowing through the emergency rooms, outpatient clinics, cafeterias, and patient account cashier windows in many hospitals is significant enough to attract even bank robber types. Some of the activities of safety and security programs that have been developed to counter such hazards include the following:

- monitoring and controlling traffic flow, both internally and externally
- providing building and grounds control and surveillance
- providing specific safety and security services to areas handling drugs, food, and monies and other departments subject to pilfering and theft
- providing patient security functions and, where necessary, assisting in restraint of unmanageable patients, families, and employees
- providing a communications link, both externally and internally, when necessary to supplement existing communications programs
- providing overall monitoring and surveillance through the use of closed-circuit television
- inspecting areas throughout the facility and recommending appropriate safety and security measures
- providing general police functions in liaison with other law enforcement and public safety agencies
- providing other appropriate functions related to safety and security

It is important to formalize safety and security services so that necessary policies, procedures, and systems can be developed to insure the most effective program. Activities designed primarily for safety and security purposes are significant risk management measures.

CORRECTIVE ACTIVITIES

Ideally, problems should never occur if all necessary preventive measures have been taken; realistically, they seem to happen despite all efforts to avoid them. The Three Laws of Murphy and other "laws of probability" seem to be proved valid over and over again.

Up until now, discussion in this chapter has centered on *preventive* activities; that is, activities designed to prevent the occurrence of problems. But what about problems that already exist?

Corrective activities need to be inventoried prior to the establishment of a risk management program. Those activities that not only remedy existing problem situations but also seek out and solve hidden or potential problems can be defined as corrective. Hopefully, corrective measures—including policies, procedures, and systems to identify, investigate, remedy, and monitor problem situations—are already an integral part of institutional operations.

Identification of Risks

The first step in correcting any risk situation is identification of the risk problem.

Though this sounds easy, two basic characteristics of human nature often deter such efforts. The first is the tendency against involvement on the part of all people. Such statements as "This is not my problem so why should I get involved in it;" "If I stop and help with this, it will only lead to a lot of trouble for me;" or "It's not my job so why should I worry about it" are common today. A second characteristic that obstructs identification of problems is the tendency of those responsible to be on the defensive. When a problem situation in a specific area is brought to the attention of someone responsible for that area, the reaction is often a defensive one. When an organization is able to overcome these two basic instincts, a healthy setting for good corrective activities is created. Attempts to emphasize corrective activities in hospitals have been successful in many cases.

Defining the cost to the organization of negative situations (for example, risk problems and resulting liability in areas of malpractice, workmen's compensation, small claims adjustment, and legal fees) can be helpful as a first step. Once these negative situations are identified, they may be interpreted to the organization in terms of the dollars which are being paid out for these negative activities rather than for *positive* ones, such as higher salaries, better fringe benefits, and improved working conditions.

Positive as well as negative reinforcement recognition in safety, loss control, and risk management activities can be built into the personnel evaluation system. This may be accomplished by incorporating questions relating to these functions in employee evaluation forms. Questions on reference inquiry forms in this area are also appropriate. Rewards and penalties must be part of the system to insure its effectiveness.

Contests among employees that emphasize safety, reporting hazards, and creating awareness of potential risk situations are a means of promoting corrective activities directed toward identification of problems. Prizes and other forms of recognition are excellent ways to create interest among the hospital staff in this approach.

"Employee interest and involvement in the loss control program is the mainspring. . . . Recognition of individual employee contributions to the safety program, and group and individual activities such as safety committees, suggestion plans, and safety campaigns will motivate interest in the program."[9]

Plant and service inspections are excellent methods of problem identification. These usually fall into two basic categories: *area* inspections and *function* inspections. The area inspection approach generally involves a tour and review of a department with the idea of identifying all problem situations, regardless of their origin. Exhibit 2–4 illustrates such an inspection format. This may be accomplished internally by the department itself, or externally by a committee or others assigned this responsibility. A functional inspection generally is conducted by a specialist seeking to define specific problems. Examples of this type of inspection might be in such areas as electrical hazards, fire prevention, and infections control.

There is always apprehension when outside inspection agencies tour the hospital on periodic licensure or regulations visits. Perhaps a better ongoing internal inspection program could be used to counter some of this apprehension and insure positive results.

Problem situations generally fall in the following categories:

- patient
- physician
- employee
- environment
- systems
- policy and procedure

Exhibit 2-4 Safety Check List

SAFETY AND LOSS CONTROL
INSPECTION REPORT

AREA _____

INSPECTED BY _____

DATE _____

Rating   S Satisfactory
Values   U Unsatisfactory

DEPARTMENT

SAFETY CHECK LIST

Checklist items:
- hallways & corridors
- stairs & stairways
- other traffic patterns
- floor surfaces
- general housekeeping
- waste receptacles
- toilet facilities
- storage
- rodent & insect control
- infectious waste control
- food preparation
- lighting
- ventilation
- temperature
- fire fighting equipment
- inspection of extinguishers
- fire doors operable
- exits (clear & marked)
- storage of flammables
- storage of medical gases
- smoking regulations enforced
- fire & disaster manuals
- emergency lighting
- electrical wiring
- condition of electrical wiring
- electrical panels, labeled
- grounding of equipment
- condition, use, extension cords
- guarding of machinery
- use of protective devices
- condition of ladders
- tools and equipment
- handling, radioactive materials
- unsafe practices

General Environment: Good | Fair | Poor

Distribution
1. — File
2. — Follow-up inspection
3. — Administration

Remarks:

Note: Report here all unsafe or unsatisfactory conditions. Continue on other side if necessary.

Source: Adaptation of form used by Kennestone Hospital, Marietta, Georgia, 1978.

Each of these categories should have an appropriate organizational mechanism to encourage identification and documentation of problem situations and referral to appropriate organizational areas for remedial action and monitoring.

Investigative Techniques

In-hospital incidents, accidents, and risk situations have been occurring since hospitals came into existence. As these things happen, organizational representatives often find themselves in the position of being "house detectives." Certain techniques should be used in the investigation process. Investigative work, whether it be something very sophisticated, like law enforcement and litigation preparation, or just basic problem solving, should follow certain principles. Such guidelines probably have not been defined *formally* in the hospital setting, but an effort to understand these in the context of corrective activities would be helpful to the organization.

When a problem is identified, certain basic steps are suggested.

1. Take care of immediate needs; provide assistance to alleviate critical situations or relieve any pressure that may exist.
2. Gather the facts; fact finding and identification are critical. Facts are differentiated from opinion in this step. This involves examination of physical evidence, obtaining reports from witnesses, establishing time elements, and a basic review of the entire situation.
3. Reconstruct the scene and situation immediately. This might involve the use of such tools as diagrams, sketches, photographs, and detailed descriptions. Log as much descriptive information as possible.
4. Determine whether the problem is part of a pattern; ask certain questions, such as: Have there been other occurrences? Does this mode of operation fit previous situations, or is this an isolated problem? Does the background of those involved relate to this problem situation in any manner? Review circumstantial evidence.
5. Identify responsibility and/or cause. Determine what and/or whom the evidence points to.
6. Build a case from the information and evidence gathered from steps 1–5 and determine an appropriate course of action.
7. Report of investigation should include the who, what, when, where, and how of the case.

As previously mentioned, such investigative techniques probably have not been formalized or even practiced very effectively in many hospitals. However, the need for them is always present. The process as part of the overall corrective activity is necessary and should be refined to insure an effective risk management program when it is established.

Remedial Action

The process of correcting a problem or eliminating a risk is probably the most important step involved in corrective activities. The main requirement to insure good remedial action within an organization is the establishment of well-defined and well-understood lines of responsibility, authority, and accountability. If one feels responsible for problem situations, has the authority to handle them, and must account for results, then effective remedial action will usually take place. *Remedial action* is problem solving; *problem solving* is decision making; and *decision making* is an active management function.

Decision-Making Process

Responsible managers involved in remedial activities have four basic courses of action available to them in the decision-making process. These are *immediate action, nonaction, deferred action,* and *restricted action.*

The first and simplest type that generally enters one's mind is *immediate action.* This course is usually necessary when time is important or when possible consequences suggest no other approach. When following this approach, the managers immediately select a positive direction in making their decisions.

If it is conscious and calculated, *nonaction,* the second alternative, is in itself an active decision. For example, an incident with potential risk ramifications occurs within a department and is brought to the attention of the responsible head. After thought and consideration, the department head decides to refrain from entering into the situation, with the feeling that it can best be resolved without intervention. In reaching such a conclusion, the manager has engaged in a mental activity or performed an administrative action and intentionally has chosen a course of nonaction.

The third course, *deferred action,* may be defined as deliberate postponement. Like nonaction, it requires a mental process but at the same time suggests another course in the future. (For example, a necessary decision to expend several thousands of dollars to eliminate a problem situation is deferred for several months until it can be budgeted in the next fiscal year.) The previous two courses should not be confused with default. The difference lies in the fact that calculated mental activity has been performed.

Restricted action, the fourth course, is the alternative selected most often, yet many times it is the least understood by a manager. This course of action fosters delegation, an important key to productive and effective management. The responsible manager restricts personal activity and places the responsibility for necessary action upon subordinates. In delegating, the manager should indicate to the subordinates what is to be done and offer guidance but should not take the challenge out of it by telling them how to do it. Let the subordinates figure it out for themselves and grow in the process.[10] In following this pattern, the manager has restricted personal activity, thus following a course of restricted action.

Some situations may require only one course of action while others require a combination of several. In such cases, combinations may be considered a fifth course.

It should be recognized that decision making as related to problem solving is necessary at all levels within the organization. However, the course of action selected will often vary from level to level. For instance, a course of restricted action at the management level relative to a given situation may lead to a course of immediate action at the supervisory level.

Default

When active decision making does not take place, passive management occurs. Passive management, better known as management by *default,* has resulted in many organizational failures. Default in this sense means forfeiting the opportunity to make decisions. It can be described as inactive or inert management, and if practiced for an extended period, it may lead the entire organizational unit into a state of inertia.

Default usually results from thoughtlessness or forgetfulness. It is often symbolized by old stacks of papers on managers' desks or in closed drawers in their credenzas. To prevent default, managers must constantly strive to be perceptive of problem situations and ramifications. If they do not, their responsibilities have been neglected.

A common failing of many managers is to ignore a problem rather than to face it and take the responsibility for attempting to solve it one way or another. After all, managers who do not make decisions can't be criticized for poor judgment. Eventually, of course, they will be criticized anyway, and for something far more serious: failing to produce results.[11]

Problem situations requiring action that for one reason or another fail to attract managers' attention may occur in day-to-day operations. In such instances, unconscious default results. Ignorance of such situations does not lessen the harmful effects that may result from a course of inactivity.

Being human, managers will from time to time be guilty of default. When this is discovered, evaluation of the situation should begin immediately and a course of action be decided upon. The situation may have remained stable. If so, action may follow the same course the initial action would have taken. However, belated action generally is more difficult because the problem situation often has deteriorated or worsened during the time interval. It may then require a defensive rather than an offensive approach, which is almost always less effective.

Red tape and bureaucratic interference can also be a deterrent to good remedial action. Administrative efforts to minimize these, particularly in the problem-solving process, will be most helpful. In general, the organization should develop a philosophy of encouraging active management that is integrated into its policies and procedures. This philosophy will foster good decision making, resulting in problem solving and, in turn, remedying risk situations.

Monitoring and Audit

The "weed theory" of problems is one that is subscribed to either consciously or unconsciously by many managers. This theory expounds that problems are like weeds; most problems are not solved, they are just cut back or mowed down only to reappear some time in the future. In other words, problems, like weeds, do not usually go away permanently; they are only eradicated after their roots are destroyed. One difficulty with this theory is that one does not know for certain that the roots are dead until a period of time has elapsed. If the weed theory is valid, then monitoring and audit systems must be applied to actions taken to remedy risk problems.

Monitoring is the last of the management processes cited earlier, and it possibly is the one practiced most poorly by managers. There exist certain monitoring techniques that, if followed, will improve and insure control of activities of problem solving. The *suspense* system is probably the most common communicative technique that results in follow-up, the key to monitoring. This system requires that courses of action be reviewed or reinstated at certain intervals through automatic reminders. It can be accomplished through a tickler file for a manager, a future agenda requirement for a committee, or a checklist item for an inspector. The Safety Inspection Followup memorandum in Exhibit 2–5 is an example of a suspense technique.

Audit, another type of review, generally is divided into two forms: internal and independent. In the context of corrective activities, both forms should be incorporated into the institution's operating systems. Internal follow-up is probably the easiest to accomplish if the responsible line managers feel the weight of responsibility and establish the suspense mechanism to insure surveillance of situations. However, an independent audit in certain problem situations can bring a more objective and constructive evaluation of the effectiveness of the problem-solving effort. Therefore, periodic reviews of departmental operations by outsiders are helpful, particularly as they relate to problem solving. The checks and balances of organizational behavior are necessary and healthy to an institution's overall well-being.

Exhibit 2-5 Safety Inspection Followup Memorandum

TO:

FROM: Safety and Loss Control Council

SUBJECT: Safety Inspection

Listed below are the findings of a recent safety inspection of your area. It is requested that you take appropriate action to resolve the correctable discrepancies.

_____

_____

_____

_____

_____

_____

_____

_____

_____

A response indicating action taken on correctable items and/or problems with noncorrectable items should be sent to the Safety and Security Department. A followup inspection will occur shortly.

_____

_____

_____

_____

_____

_____

_____

_____

_____

_____

_____

                                   _____
                                          Department Head

Source: Adaptation of form used by Kennestone Hospital, Marietta, Georgia, 1978.

The most recent additions to the institutional monitoring process are patient care audits. With impetus provided by the JCAH, medical and nursing audits are being incorporated into the objective criteria for evaluation of patient care, which are replacing the almost totally subjective criteria previously used. According to current JCAH standards,

> ... there shall be continuous monitoring, with enforcement, of those elements of patient care identified in the medical staff or clinical department/service rules and regulations .... Evidence of the quality of patient care provided in the hospital shall be demonstrated by measurement of actual care against criteria .... Criteria must be explicit and measurable, and must reflect the optimal level of care that can be achieved through current medical and related health science knowledge ....[12]

and additionally,

> The quality of care provided by the nursing staff shall be measured as part of the hospital's patient care evaluation program ....[13]

Monitoring and auditing functions in both patient and nonpatient care areas, serve as primary corrective activities within a hospital. Continuous evaluation of the actions of the entire organization and of its component parts tends to create a more risk-free environment.

DOCUMENTARY ACTIVITIES

The quality of services provided in a hospital is generally judged by audit and evaluation committees, accrediting agencies, licensure bodies, and even by the courts through documented records. The task of writing or recording actions at all levels is one of the most important internal functions within a hospital. Often the performance of this task is looked upon, particularly by professionals, as menial, without purpose, and an interference with more pressing responsibilities. A common statement by physicians is, "My job is to treat patients and not to do all the paper work for the hospital." One can feel some sympathy for this attitude, given the multiple forms and records that are necessary today. Certainly, effort should be made to alleviate unnecessary paper work and provide clerical support when possible to handle some of these duties. However, one must never forget that the *record* is crucial, not only from a quality but also from a continuity standpoint.

An inventory of necessary recordkeeping and documentary activities that must be performed includes the following items:

1. Patient and medical records
2. Governing body records
   a. Bylaws
   b. Minutes and reports
3. Medical staff records
   a. Bylaws, rules and regulations
   b. Credential records
   c. Minutes and reports
4. Personnel records
5. Financial records
   a. Purchasing records
   b. Financial audits and reports
   c. Patient accounts
   d. Budgets
6. Written policies and procedures
   a. General policy
   b. Interdepartmental (Standard Policies and Procedures)
   c. Intradepartmental (Departmental Policies and Procedures)
   d. Personnel (Personnel Policies and Procedures)
7. Administrative records
   a. Contracts
   b. Deeds and trusts
   c. Correspondence
8. Regulatory Reports
   a. Accreditation surveys
   b. Licensure surveys
   c. Other agency reports
9. Quality assurance reports
   a. Medical
   b. Nonmedical
10. Risk management and loss control records

Number 10 will be reviewed in detail later, but it should be noted here that many documentary records and reports that will fit into a formal risk management program currently exist in most hospitals.

EDUCATIONAL ACTIVITIES

Education is the hospital's strongest tool for maintaining and improving the quality of care it delivers. In a liability control system, the role of education becomes even more critical, and potentially more rewarding.[14]

Education is a function of the governing body, the administration, the medical staff, and every department of a hospital. For many years JCAH has required ongoing educational programs in all areas of operation. For example, the JCAH *Accreditation Manual* contains the following statements.

> The potential effectiveness of the governing body is indicated by . . . a program for the orientation and continuing education of governing body members . . . .
> There shall be a program of continuing medical education designed to keep the medical staff informed of significant new developments and new skills in medicine. Medical staff education should include hospital based activities as well as educational opportunities available outside of the hospital . . . .
> There shall be continuing training programs and educational opportunities for the development of nursing personnel . . . .[15]

Staff Education

Many hospitals have educational service departments, as well as departmental activities relating to education. This centralization enhances and supplements departmental efforts and allows interdisciplinary educational activities to be developed, coordinated, and presented.

In addition to providing educational opportunities, it is important to document all education and training activities. Permanent records of all education and training programs attended by individual hospital personnel (both in the hospital and away from it) that may serve as criteria in the evaluation of individual performance should be maintained.

Formal programs should be offered both in the technical aspects of the individual job and in interpersonal relations and supervisory and administrative skills where appropriate. Programs directed at motivation and self-actualization also have an important place in the hospital's educational activities.

A specific example in this regard might prove helpful.

> Kennestone Hospital's motto, *Professionally We Serve, Personally We Care* has instilled a feeling of responsibility among employees to continue to update their knowledge and skills to provide quality patient services. In order to provide the numerous programs requested by all staff levels, the Hospital has maintained an active department of educational services, with full administrative support.
> It is the philosophy of the department that the learning process is continuous and extends throughout the life of the productive individual. Continuing one's education leads to a feeling of self

actualization and becomes a key in motivation of employees and resultant job satisfaction. If people feel good about themselves, this positive attitude is transferred in interactions with patients, families and other staff members.

Perhaps one of the most meaningful attitudinal programs offered by the department is the human relations course which was developed and is taught inhouse by the hospital's Educational Services Staff Development Coordinator, and Mental Health Unit Staff Coordinator.

The goal of the course is to enable staff members to deal more effectively with the barriers which obstruct and hinder positive relationships with families, patients and fellow employees.

The program consists of six sessions lasting two hours each. Course content includes:

Session I	Introduction and Transactional Analysis Theory
Session II	Introduction of Communication Theory Factors Which Influence Communication
Session III	Keys to Effective Communication
Session IV	Language Approaches to More Effective Communication, Indirect and Direct Communication
Session V	Problem Solving and Gaming
Session VI	Work Related Conflict Resolution Summary, Discussion and Evaluation

In an effort to offer the quality of staff development programs that was desired, the majority of offerings were submitted to local colleges or universities for approval for Continuing Education Units (CEU's) and/or to the State Nurses Association for review by the Continuing Education Approval and Recognition Program (CEARP).

Recognition received by the employees through these agencies has had a direct and positive effect upon the improvement of patient services.

Any programs which are developed to reinforce positive employee attitudes are not without pitfalls. It is therefore important that they be continually reevaluated and change various aspects to ensure that they meet the ever changing needs of personnel in the institution which will result in improved patient services.

Perhaps the best method to measure the effect of human relations offerings is the positive responses received on the patient services questionnaire and the personnel turnover rate which remains among the lowest.[16]

Patient Education

Formal patient education is another activity that has become more prevalent in hospitals in recent years. The need for patients to understand their diseases and/or injuries and the diagnostic and treatment methods to be used is very important. Additionally, patient education assists significantly in pre- and post-hospital care. Better informed and more knowledgeable patients tend to be more satisfied with their therapy and to develop more positive attitudes toward the institution and its staff.

Well-qualified, -trained, and -motivated staff may be one of the best risk prevention assets a hospital can have. Education programs directed toward these purposes are essential.

According to Barry A. Passett, the education function has three critical roles to play in the success of a liability control system.

- The first is the traditional one of providing staff training and patient education . . . .
- The second role is to orient the hospital and medical staffs to the liability control system and to conduct skills training in the various components of the system.
- The third role of education is to be responsive, through the continuing education of the nursing and medical staffs, to deficiencies that are disclosed through nursing audit, medical audit, and other quality assurance/liability control procedures.[17]

ADMINISTRATIVE ACTIVITIES

The administrative framework that sustains operational programs within a hospital is extremely important to the success of risk management. For maximum results, the involvement of all administrative levels is essential. This involvement must be accompanied by an understanding throughout the organization that administration is an active process that requires judgment and communication to create forward motion toward institutional goals. Additionally, all administrative activities must be guided by operating principles that encourage ethical conduct, consistency, and purpose in the organization's efforts.

To insure a common understanding of the role of administration, an administrative philosophy should be developed within an organization. The technique used by this author to accomplish this difficult task is the use of administrative policy memoranda that are distributed to the hospital's administrative staff, including department heads. The following related thoughts are summarized from these documents and attempt to place administrative activities in a context that will be supportive of such hospital programs as risk management.

The Department Head's Role

Often the administrator or chief executive officer is thought to *be* the administration of an organization. This is true only in one case: a one-person organization. Administration must be a function of the entire organization if its true effect is to be felt. Department heads (and supervisors) are a significant part of administration and, therefore, must also be administrators.

Department heads in such institutions as hospitals generally find that they must acquire at least two types of knowledge to be effective. The first is the *technical* knowledge of the departmental specialty. Knowledge of nursing skills for a director of nursing, of technological skills for a chief technologist, and of housekeeping and sanitation for an executive housekeeper are examples. The other type is the *administrative* knowledge that must be possessed by department heads to get the job done through those working under and with them. Most individuals who reach the department head level in a given field have been adequately trained or have adequate experience in the technical knowledge of the job. Many times, however, they have received little or no exposure to the administrative knowledge demanded by the position. In short, department heads must not only be specialists in their fields, but be administrators as well.

How does one acquire administrative knowledge? Most humans are creatures of habit. Department heads must study and practice the skills of administration until they become habit and can be performed almost without even thinking about what is taking place. This principle became clear while viewing a demonstration by a collegiate coach who was explaining the art of shooting a basketball. He instructed his players to go through the act of holding and shooting the ball over and over with no intention of ringing the goal. He explained that it was important that a player develop the mechanics of shooting to a point where they became habit, or automatic. Once this is accomplished, the player can concentrate on putting the ball into the basket.

The same holds true for administration. Initially, it is a process of constant concentration on the fundamental functions of management. After such practice, individuals soon find themselves performing the functions automatically. It should be noted, however, that administrative knowledge does not remain static, and efforts must be made to keep pace with new developments and to change administrative habits whenever appropriate.

What are these management functions that are important for the success of department heads? They are defined in many ways by many different authorities in the field. The following functions are generally acceptable to most authorities: planning, organizing, directing, coordinating, and monitoring. Instead of dwelling in detail on these functions, attention will be directed to an important underlying factor involved in each: decision making.

Administration as an Active Process

To act or not to act? This is a question many department heads ask themselves when faced with day-to-day decisions affecting their department. If administration is to fulfill its proper role, there is but one answer to this question; administration must always act. As one author said, "All progress flows through man's mind in action.[18]"

What is this phenomenon called action and why is it important in administration? It may be simply defined as the doing of something; the state of being in motion or working.[19] As such, action becomes a vital part of a modern organization. Administration must generate action that creates organizational movement toward predetermined goals. As certain courses of action are examined, it will become evident that administration must be active if an organization is to succeed.

Need for Judgment

In any situation, before making a decision or selecting a course of action, an administrator should demand the *facts* relative to the particular situation. The degree of availability of facts on which courses of action will be based is inversely related to the extent to which judgment must be used in determining action. Adequate quantity and quality of facts will usually suggest and may even dictate a certain course of action. Lack of facts will necessitate the use of judgment. According to the late Ray Brown in his book, *Judgment in Administration,* most administrative problems are problems only because the full facts are not known.[20] As once stated by Samuel Butler, "Life is the art of drawing sufficient conclusions from insufficient premises."

Some administrators theorize that success results from a high percentage of good judgments made in the decision-making process. For example, those who make 60–70 percent good decisions that are based on their judgment are assured of success. This seems somewhat farfetched, for the other 30–40 percent may be the most crucial and important decisions affecting attainment of organizational objectives. In this case, an administrator, though boasting a high batting average, could be sitting the game out on the bench or even be back in the minor leagues.

Judgment is needed both in determining appropriate courses of action and in deciding which situations require personal attention and careful consideration. Certain situations do not require deep and perceptive thought on the part of persons at the executive level; they may be insignificant or they may and should be handled by lower echelons within the organization. Individuals should be cognizant of their positions within the organizational hierarchy. They should utilize their time and energies at the level that is most beneficial to the organization.

Here, again, it should be emphasized that administrative action in decision making should be a process used at all organizational levels, not just by the executive echelon.

Communications as a Form of Action

Administrative action many times takes the form of communication. It is often said that administrators do not do much themselves; they just see that someone gets it done. Action is achieved through communication of instructions.[21] Communication is the tool often used to activate a selected course.

A quarterback selects and calls the plays in the huddle so that all members of the football team will know their assignments when the ball is snapped. Why bother to select a course of action if it is not to be followed by the organizational team?

Motion in Organization

Action in administration generates *motion,* which is important for organizational progress. An organization should have defined objectives. To reach these, it must move *forward;* objectives are always ahead. An environment of motion is most favorable to reaching objectives. This environment can be described as a psychological attitude within the organization; it is a *feeling* of movement and progress. Occurrences in the sports' world are prime examples of this attitude.

On the fifteenth tee in the final round of the 1966 U.S. Open Golf Championship, Arnold Palmer, leading by five strokes, was aiming toward the Open record held by the great Ben Hogan. He double bogeyed the hole, which his playing partner in second place, Billy Casper, birdied. Casper subsequently tied Palmer, necessitating a playoff, which Casper ultimately won. After the round, Palmer, while being questioned by a reporter, stated, "I started thinking about shooting a 274 (the record) and that's when I made my first mistake . . . . When we'd finished the fifteenth, I began to wonder. I knew what could happen, and that's what happened."

Motion was retarded and the psychological attitude toward the objective changed, resulting in defeat rather than victory.

Dan Custes stated it very aptly, "Our success or our failure is the result of our mental condition, our thoughts about people and about ourselves, our attitudes toward people and toward ourselves."

To perpetuate necessary motion, an organization must have well-defined short-range as well as long-range objectives. Motion toward objectives will continue only if a sense of accomplishment can be attained by individuals within the organization. Lower echelons often will not realize how they are contributing to long-range goals, but they can see and understand the short-range ones as they are accomplished. Long-range objectives are also necessary tools, for they provide direction for the short-range objectives.

The space program of the 1960s had the long-range objective of landing men on the moon and returning them safely to earth. There were also short-range objectives in the program for the accomplishment of certain steps, such as rendezvous, docking, spacewalking, and soft lunar landing. All of these were necessary for the success of the ultimate manned flight to the moon. Each success resulted in jubilant enthusiasm and the desire to take the next step forward.

It is the responsibility of an organization and of administration in its leadership role to generate motion through action. Chester Barnard, in discussing the *Theory of Opportunism,* stated ". . . in most cases the ends of organizational action are the unique results of the *action* of the organization itself."[22]

Action Based on Principles

The foregoing comments were not intended to imply that action should be indiscriminate. Indiscriminate action may be more detrimental to organizational progress than default or omission of action. Any action taken should be based on the operating management *principles* of an administrator or decision maker.

Principles in administration are rules of conduct on which action is based. Adherence to these rules will result in action that is consistent and purposeful. Abraham Lincoln once stated, "Important principles may and must be inflexible."

Previous emphasis has been placed on the fact that conscious, deliberate thought is a part of the decision-making process. Decision makers, if trained to constantly direct their *thinking* toward the attainment of goals of the organization, will be in a better position to insure organizational progress. Here again judgment is often the keynote in making determinations as to which administrative action is best for a given situation.

In recapping administrative activity, what does all this mean? Department heads (and supervisors) must be administrators. They must not only be well acquainted with technical skills but also with administrative functions involved in managing their departments.

Most importantly, as administrators they must be active decision makers. When faced with situations (and they should seek out the situations that need to be faced), they will ask this question: What should be done? Then, after conscious deliberate thought, they will decide what should be done and do it!

The purpose of active rather than passive administration is to create motion–organizational motion toward objectives and goals. Calculated conscious action is always better than default, provided the action is based on administrative principles. Action taken today will often prevent situations tomorrow that will require *reaction* from a less strategic position for an administrator.

Activity or inertia, action or default, these are the choices that will often make the difference between organizational success or failure.[23]

In the context of risk management, as in any organizational endeavor, administrative activity cannot be emphasized enough. Administration exists to accomplish organizational purposes; therefore, effective administration is necessary for the success of any new program.

CONCLUSION

Thus far, discussion in this chapter has concerned five basic categories of organizational activities that are prerequisites for establishment of a risk management program: preventive, corrective, documentary, educational, and administrative activities. Obviously, all of these prerequisites will not exist in every hospital. Conducting an organizational inventory prior to the establishment of a formal risk management program will serve a useful purpose.

All of the organizational activities cited will in time become a part of the risk management program itself. In other words, preventive, corrective, documentary, educational, and administrative activities are not only functions which *should* exist prior to the implementation of risk management, they are activities that *must* exist as integral parts of the program as it develops within the hospital structure. At the same time, risk management, if it serves its rightful purpose, will reinforce the other operational functions. A healthy interdependence will be likely to develop among all related activities. Such is the way a new functional member should be welcomed into an organizational family.

RISK MANAGEMENT PREREQUISITES CHECKLIST

Preventive activities

___ Do you have a patient relations program?

___ Do you have a patient representative program?

___ Do you have a means of immediately handling patient complaints?

___ Do you have family support and involvement programs?

___ Do you have a patient service questionnaire and are its results distributed?

___ Do you have a community or public relations program?

___ Is an individual responsible for public relations?

___ Do you have an active media relations program?

___ Does your hospital have means for community input?

___ Does it have public representatives on the governing body?

___ Are hospital representatives involved in community activities?

___ Do you have an effective volunteer program?

___ Do you have a personnel relations program?

___ Do you have an effective personnel and employment department?

___ Does a healthy family atmosphere exist in the hospital?

___ Do you have a hospital slogan, credo, or written purpose?

___ Do you have an administrative personnel exchange program?

___ Does your hospital have an employee recognition program?

___ Do you have an employee newsletter?

___ Do you have a medical staff relations program?

___ Do physicians serve on the governing body?

___ Do effective medical staff-hospital liaison activities exist?

___ Does your hospital have a medical director or director of medical affairs?

___ Do you have a medical staff secretary?

___ Do you have a medical staff newsletter?

___ Do you conduct a periodic medical staff opinion poll?

___ Are hospital representatives on medical staff committees?

___ Do you have an active environmental services program?

___ Do you have a preventive maintenance program?

___ Do you have an adequate groundskeeping program?

___ Do quality control programs for environmental services exist?

___ Do you have medical equipment mechanics and/or biomedical engineers on your staff?

___ Are zone maintenance and housekeeping programs in operation?

___ Do you have ongoing project planning, coordination, and review functions?

___ Do you have a formal safety and security program?

___ Is a safety and security director on your staff?

___ Do you have a surveillance system for facilities and grounds?

___ Do you conduct regular safety and security inspection programs?

___ Does good liaison with local law enforcement and public safety agencies exist?

Corrective activities

___ Do you encourage problem identification?

___ Do programs including rewards and recognition to encourage staff involvement exist?

___ Are contests held to identify potential risk problems?

___ Do you have area inspection programs?

___ Do you have functional inspection programs?

___ Are problem situations remedied expeditiously in your hospital?

___ Do managers within the organization know how to solve problems?

___ Does red tape deter good decision making?

___ Are incentives provided to good problem solvers?

___ Is there an attitude prevalent of not wanting to get involved?

___ Are responsible managers overly defensive to constructive criticism?

___ Are problem situations monitored in your hospital?

___ Do you have suspense systems to assist in the follow-up?

___ Do internal audit functions exist in all areas?

___ Are systems of independent audit available?

Documentary activities

___ Are good records a part of ongoing hospital operations?

___ Are patient and medical records adequate?

___ Are governing body and medical staff records adequate?

___ Are personnel records adequate?

___ Are administrative and financial records adequate?

___ Are policies and procedures recorded?

___ Are regulatory reports maintained and referenced?

___ Are quality assurance records adequate?

___ Are records and reports dealing with potential risk and loss adequately maintained?

Educational activities

___ Are educational activities a part of ongoing hospital operations?

___ Are educational functions handled on an intradepartmental basis?

___ Do you have an educational services department?

___ Are records of educational activities maintained?

___ Are personal as well as technical skills included in educational programs?

___ Do you have a patient education program?

Administrative activities

___ Has administrative philosophy been formalized in your hospital?

___ Is administration a front-office function only?

___ Are department heads administrators?

___ Is administration an active process in your hospital?

Note: This checklist is not meant to be all-inclusive nor does it require absolute adherence. Its purpose is to stimulate thought and redirect attitudes toward the establishment of a risk management program.

NOTES

1. S. Holloway and A. Sax, "AHA Urges, Aids Hospitals to Adopt Effective Risk Management Plans," *Hospitals, JAHA,* May 16, 1977, p. 57.

2. T. Chittenden, "Role of Physician in Malpractice Needs More Careful Exploration," *Hospitals, JAHA,* May 16, 1977, p. 53.

3. "Medical Malpractice: Is the Crisis Over?" *Consumer Representative,* September 1977, p. 544.

4. A. Sax, "Patient Advocate Programs Gain Support," *Malpractice Digest,* May/June 1977, p. 4.

5. Helen Yura and Mary B. Walsh, *The Nursing Process* (New York, N.Y.: Appleton-Century-Crofts, 1973), p. 1.

6. B. Brown and L. McFarland, "Good Employee Relations Programs Do Improve Patient Services," *Cross-References on Resources Management,* January/February 1978, pp. 7–8.

7. B. Brown, "The Profession of Hospital Administration," *Southern Hospitals,* February 1969, p. 14.

8. B. Brown, "Staff Opinion Polls," *Hospitals, JAHA,* June 16, 1970, p. 70.

9. G. Newman, "Basic Elements of a Loss Control Program," *Hospital Progress,* November 1974, p. 48.

10. From *Management Memos* (West Orange, N.J.: The Economic Press, Inc., 1965).

11. Ibid.

12. *Accreditation Manual for Hospitals* (Chicago, Ill.: Joint Commission on Accreditation of Hospitals, 1978), pp. 85, 131.

13. Ibid, p. 96.

14. B. Passett, "Education Can Help Control Hospital Liability," *Cross-References,* May/June 1977, p. 7.

15. *Accreditation Manual for Hospitals* (Chicago, Ill.: Joint Commission on Accreditation of Hospitals, 1976), pp. 76, 112, 124.

16. Brown and McFarland, pp. 8–9.

17. Passett, p. 10.

18. W. Peterson, *This Week Magazine,* October 28, 1962, p. 2.

19. *Webster's New World Dictionary of the American Language* (Cleveland: The World Publishing Company, 1960), p. 7.

20. Ray E. Brown, *Judgment in Administration* (New York: McGraw-Hill Book Company, 1966), p. 120.

21. Victor Lazzaro, *Systems and Procedures: A Handbook for Business and Industry* (Englewood Cliffs, N.J.: Prentice-Hall, Inc., 1960), p. 102.

22. Chester I. Barnard, *The Functions of the Executive* (Cambridge, Mass.: Harvard University Press, 1938), p. 200.

23. B. Brown, "Department Heads Are Also Administrators," Administrative Philosophy Memorandum, 1975, unpublished.

Chapter 3

Organization of a Risk Management Program

The establishment of a risk management program within the hospital organizational structure may be accomplished in numerous ways. Regardless of the form that the program ultimately takes, certain guidelines relating to its inception should be taken into consideration.

1. A risk management program should be coordinated with and enhance existing programs and organizational activities.
2. Risk management is basically a staff function, the purpose of which is to advise and support other operational activities of the organization.
3. The risk management program should be broad in scope to impact all departments within the hospital.
4. There must be adequate commitment in terms of management, manpower, methods, materials, and money to insure success of the program.
5. A risk management program, given time and support, should carry its own weight and justify its own existence from both service and fiscal standpoints.

The review of existing programs emphasized in Chapter 2 sets the stage for the establishment of a risk management program. Coordination, redirection, and enhancement of these programs is an excellent beginning point. To some degree all existing hospital activities should be involved in risk management. Mechanisms to provide input and feedback from both directions need to be incorporated into the organizational structure established for the program. Much of this interchange can be accomplished through developing cooperative attitudes among the managers of the different departments. Additionally, formal methods should also be established through policies, procedures, operational systems, and committee functions.

The risk management function logically fits within the definition of a *staff* rather than a *line* service. In this context, a staff service is described as supporting or advising in nature. The true purpose of a risk management program is to support and advise the entire organization in problems or situations that may pose risks to patients, public, staff, or the organization in general. Figure 3-1 shows this line and staff functional relationship relative to the risk management program.

The risk management function, like other organizational activities, must be given adequate support to fulfill its purpose. Any program must have a commitment from top administrative levels, and this must be accompanied by the manpower, methods, materials, and money necessary to insure success.

Though all of these components are necessary, possibly the most crucial is management support. A loss-control program will be successful only if a hospital's administration is convinced of the need for such a program. The administrator must assume an interest and a positive role in the development and administration of the program. The administrator's interest in the program almost invariably will be reflected in the attitudes of all members of the supervisory force, and employees' attitudes will reflect those of their supervisors. If the hospital's administrator is not interested in preventing

Figure 3-1 Hospital Organization Chart: Line and Staff Functions

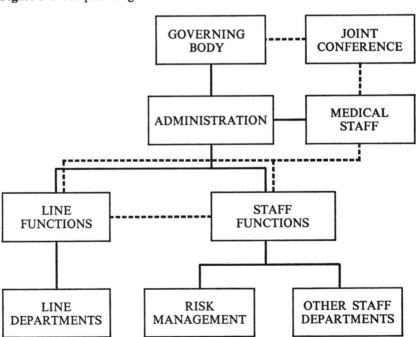

accidents and injuries, no one in the hospital will be concerned about the problem.[1]

If a risk management program does not result in a reduction of losses and does not improve services in general through the avoidance of risk problems, then the formalization of such a function is questionable. Chapter 5 will be devoted entirely to the feasibility and justification of a risk management program.

ROLE OF THE RISK MANAGER

The initiation of any new program generally starts with the designation of a manager or director who will accept operational responsibility and take the ball and run with it. Risk management is no different. If the program is to be a serious and effective activity, it will require the direction of a manager.

At this point, some of the questions which come to mind relative to a risk manager are: Is this a full-time job? How much will we have to pay for someone to handle this? What kind of person do we need? In looking at these and other related questions, each organization must individually decide which direction it wishes to follow. The current needs and problems in the area of risk prevention and loss control must be taken into consideration as well as the existing environment relative to potential litigation within the local community. The size and scope of institutional activities and the resources available also influence the hospital's decisions in regard to this program. It should be remembered that for any activity to get off the ground, effective leadership is necessary from some source.

In attempting to answer some of the above questions and to determine the type of individual required, an institution should probably follow the format most often used in the establishment of any other new program. In this regard, an organization usually starts slowly and allows growth and expansion of the program to occur as effectiveness and positive impact grow.

A conservative approach might be to initiate the position of risk manager on a part-time basis and to develop it into a full-time responsibility as needed. A variation of this approach might be to expand an existing job to take the additional responsibility rather than establishing the new function independently. Again, these are basic decisions that must be made by individual hospitals.

Most current risk managers' backgrounds and training are in hospital administration, insurance, or safety engineering. The majority were also employed by their hospitals prior to assuming responsibility for risk management activities. Their earlier experience frequently included positions in the area of hospital finance, personnel, research, education, safety, nursing, security, and claims management.[2]

Developing the Position

In developing the role of risk manager, certain factors should be taken into consideration, irrespective of which direction the organization takes relative to the above decisions.

1. Since the function is generally new to an organization and broad in nature, *proved* leadership should be provided when selecting the risk manager. If a new individual is employed, care should be taken to recruit one who has strengths in organizational development, creativeness, interpersonal relations, and persuasive abilities and who is generally a self-starter. If someone already in the organization is given this responsibility, credentials certainly should include proved skills such as these. It is clear that the benefits derived for the organization through its risk management program are largely contingent on the risk manager's innovativeness and intraorganizational planning ability.[3]
2. The title *risk manager* or some appropriate designation should be given to the one in charge of this program to establish identity. This is important because new programs many times lack ability to operate effectively unless necessary emphasis is given, a distinct entity is created, and visibility is established.[4] If the individual also has other responsibilities, this title of risk manager should be incorporated in the existing title (e.g., Director of Safety, Security, and Loss Prevention; Director of Personnel and Risk Manager; Assistant Administrator for Environmental Services and Risk Management).
3. The most appropriate organizational location for the risk manager is on the *staff* side of the chart. If the risk management function is to be incorporated into an existing position, the staff activities inherent with the position could possibly be handled more effectively by one already having staff responsibilities. This certainly does not mean that this program could not effectively fit in a *line* department or division of the organization, but it must be primarily recognized as a staff function.
4. It is important to recognize the fact that the risk manager will be coming into contact with persons at all levels within the organization because of the broad nature of activities involved in this function. Discussions related to professional activities with a nurse, analysis of a report with a data processor, the investigation of an incident with a housekeeping assistant, or a planning conference with an administrator may all be part of the day-to-day activities of the risk manager. Therefore, a need will exist to have a risk manager who is capable of handling diverse and varying activities.

5. As soon as justification exists, the position of risk manager should become a full-time position to insure adequate commitment and interest in developing the full potential of the program.
6. A job description and classification should clearly spell out the responsibilities, duties, and requirements of the position and its relationship with other activities and functions in the organization. An adequate salary with accompanying fringe benefits should be established to attract the level of person necessary to direct this important function.

Job Description

The job description of the risk manager will need to be developed to meet the needs and expectations of the individual hospital. Certain basic functions should be included, as in the example that follows.

Job Description—Risk Manager
(Example)

Title—Director of Safety, Security, and Loss Prevention
Occupational summary:

- Coordinate all aspects and perform activities related to security, safety, and risk identification, evaluation, and treatment within the hospital.
- Analyze and investigate actual as well as potential risks in the institution.
- Establish operational procedures, programs, and other methods to avoid, reduce, or minimize losses.

Work performed:

- Develop and maintain a system for the proper reporting, follow-up investigation, analysis, and file of all incidents that occur on hospital property.
- Responsible for aspects of Workmen's Compensation as directed by Occupational Safety and Health Act and Workmen's Compensation laws; work closely with Personnel Department in regard to these activities.
- Serve as Chairman of the Safety and Loss Control Council. Participate in other committees that deal with potential loss situations.
- Select, train, and assign security/safety personnel according to indicated protection requirements.
- Perform fire marshal and disaster coordinator activities related to the

hospital; work closely with related committees in regard to these activities.

- Maintain a key control system to meet the hospital's security needs.
- Confer with hospital management and staff to formulate policies and procedures relating to security and loss prevention. Interpret these policies and direct subordinates in their enforcement.
- Direct periodic inspections of the hospital facility to achieve compliance of governing regulatory agencies' requirements. Report discrepancies to the appropriate authority for corrective action.
- Conduct security audits to determine loss vulnerabilities within departmental operations. Consult with the hospital's legal counsel on matters of potential liability. Review loss-prevention methods with management and staff to assure compliance.
- Assist appropriate departments and committees in periodic review of all release and consent forms and procedures to assure necessary hospital/patient understanding and agreement regarding the treatment or procedural information to be provided.
- Advise and assist the Claims Management Committee in regard to handling of claims, including adjusting.
- Assist in quality assurance activities throughout the hospital as they relate to the risk management function.

Education, knowledge and ability:

- College degree with one year of related experience or an associate degree with three years of related experience. Training in hospital security, safety, and loss prevention. Ability to effectively supervise and direct the work of others.
- Considerable knowledge of law enforcement and investigation techniques. Ability to work cooperatively with hospital management and local law enforcement agencies. Ability to apply judgment and discretion in handling confidential information.

Risk managers have been employed by hospitals only recently, and in many instances their responsibilities and functions are still being defined and described.[5] Experts in the field agree that the risk manager who implements and coordinates the hospital's risk management program, should be a member of the hospital's administrative team.[6] There is also general agreement that the risk manager must have the active support of the hospital's governing board, administration, medical staff, and all employees, especially the nursing staff, if the job activities are to be successfully carried out.[7]

STRUCTURING A PROGRAM

In developing an effective risk management program, the process of successfully integrating existing activities with new functions is essential but it need not be complicated. In examining current activities, particularly relating to the handling of risk situations, one will find much being performed by committees. Therefore, an ideal starting place for structuring the risk management program is the committee organization. Coordination, redirection, and expansion, in certain cases of these existing committee activities, will be necessary in this regard. The related committees will generally fall into two basic categories: first, safety and loss control; second, quality assurance.

Some of these committee functions currently existing in most hospitals include security, safety, disaster planning, infections control, environmental control, education, patient care evaluation, and others. Generally, hospital committees have functioned somewhat independently while fulfilling their respective purposes. Organizationally, they normally fit jurisdictionally in departments or divisions that have operational responsibilities relative to the committees' functions (e.g., patient safety as a part of the nursing or patient services division, employee safety as a part of the personnel department, fire safety as a part of the engineering department, patient care evaluation as part of the medical staff). At times, such committees have been developed solely to meet specific accreditation standards, licensure regulations, or insurance requirements and, because of this, lack real purpose and effectiveness.

Safety and Loss Control

The number, names, and composition of committees relating to safety and loss control will vary among hospitals, but the purposes and objectives of these committees are generally similar.

In structuring the risk management program, an effort to revitalize, if necessary, the functions of these related committees will be helpful. It is equally as important that these activities be integrated to achieve maximum effectiveness. The functions and activities of one committee often relate to or overlap those of another. For example, unsafe environmental situations that endanger patients may also be hazardous to personnel, and the functions related to correcting these may fall under the jurisdiction of two different committees. The risk management program can serve as the means by which related committee efforts are centralized and coordinated. A suggested council/committee structure (Figure 3-2) related to these activities that attempts to accomplish this integration follows.

Figure 3-2 Risk Management Council/Committee Structure

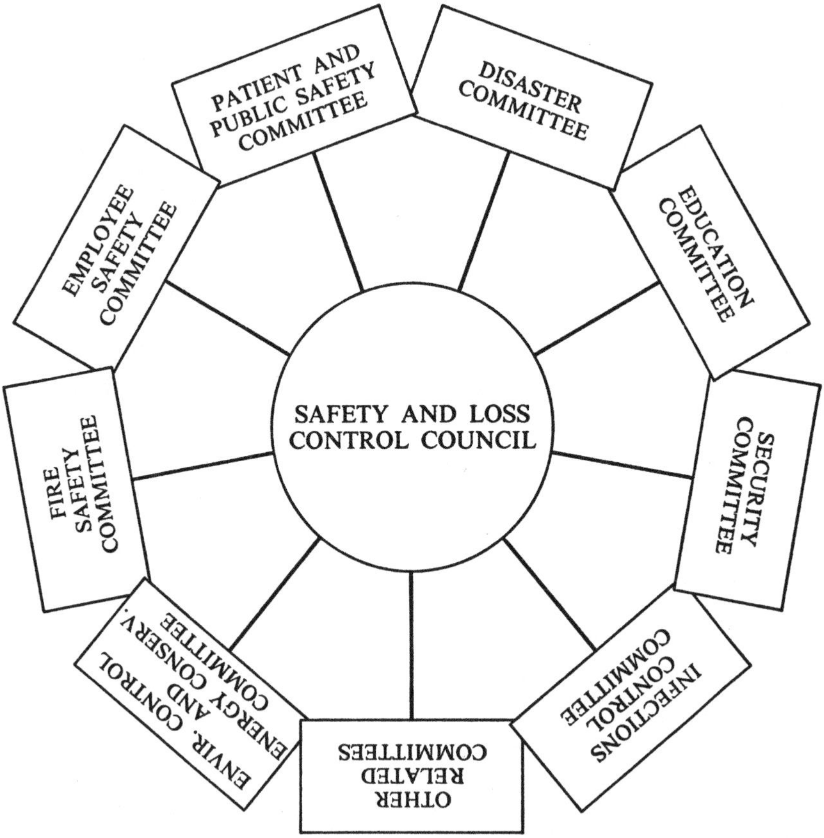

Safety and Loss Control Council

This council is composed of multiple committees having specific responsibilities for different aspects of the risk management program. It includes committees such as:

1. *Environment Control and Energy Conservation:* conducts facility inspections and develops policies and procedures relative to the provision of a safe and comfortable environment while attempting to conserve energy resources.
2. *Fire safety:* coordinates and monitors fire drills and reviews critiques of

these drills. Reviews and updates the fire and internal disaster plan and develops policies and procedures relative to fire safety.

3. *Employee Safety:* reviews all accident reports and makes recommendations for appropriate action. Develops policies and procedures relative to employee safety.

4. *Patient and Public Safety:* reviews all incident reports and makes recommendations for appropriate action. Develops policies and procedures relative to patient and public safety.

5. *Disaster:* coordinates and monitors disaster drills and reviews critiques of drills. Reviews and updates disaster plan and develops policies and procedures relative to the handling of an external disaster.

6. *Education:* conducts orientation and training programs to support the hospital's overall safety program. Coordinates these activities with other educational efforts.

7. *Security:* reviews all incident/accident reports that have security implications and makes recommendations for appropriate action. Develops policies and procedures relative to security in and around the hospital.

8. *Infections Control:* reviews and monitors the infection control program and recommends appropriate action. Develops policies and procedures relative to infections control throughout the hospital.

9. *Other:* related committees can be added as needed.

It should be noted that this council/committee structure is only an example. Whatever configuration the committee takes, an equitable balance of department head, supervisory, and nonsupervisory membership is desirable. (See Appendix B for suggested composition.)

A system of rotating and periodically replacing nonpermanent members may be used to insure broad representation as well as the resulting educational benefits. It is amazing how balanced representation, periodic changes in membership, and broad involvement can vitalize committee functions. For example, a nonsupervising nurse who has worked in an emergency room where victims of a plane crash or an industrial explosion have been treated may be immensely more knowledgeable and interested in the Disaster Committee than someone in an administrative office who has been isolated from many of the direct care activities involved in such situations.

Employee interest and involvement in the loss control program is the mainspring, as in any program. Without this interest and involvement, the most carefully planned program simply will not work.[8]

Quality Assurance

In the AHA manual entitled *Quality Assurance Program for Medical Care in the Hospital,* the question "Why Quality Assurance Programs?" is asked. Here is a portion of the answer.

> The advances of medicine in the Twentieth Century have provided mankind with the capability to cure many diseases and control the course of others. The capability has changed the right of access to quality medical services from a luxury to a utilitarian necessity in today's world. It has given society as a group and the community as individuals a justifiable role in determining how, when, where, and what medical services should be delivered. Further, it has given the patient who receives care and those who purchase care for him (third party payers, government, employers, unions, and so forth) a right to the assurance that care received is of optimal quality.[9]

As emphasized previously, quality patient care and risk management are distinctly related and compatible, and this interdependence should be recognized by the hospital's governing body, administration, and professional staff.[10] Numerous committees exist in most hospitals that have as their primary objective the assurance of quality service. Some of these that relate to the risk management function include:

1. *Professional Committee of the Governing Body,* which

   - becomes directly involved in the approval of medical staff privileges and related disciplinary actions;
   - reviews medical and nursing audits and participates in other patient care evaluation procedures;
   - reviews any changes in medical staff bylaws, rules, and regulations; and
   - makes recommendations to the governing body concerning such matters.

2. *Joint Conference and Accreditation Committee,* which

   - handles intercommunications between the governing body, medical staff, and administration;
   - monitors compliance with standards set by the JCAH.

3. *Medical Staff Committees,* which

- develop requirements for membership and delineation of privileges;
- organize the medical staff;
- evaluate professional qualifications and performance;
- conduct functions relating to patient care and promote programs of continuing professional education. (Committee functions are enumerated later in this chapter under Medical Staff Committees)

4. *Nursing Committee,* which

- continuously evaluates policies, procedures, and practices relative to nursing care rendered in the hospital.

5. *Education Committee,* which

- provides hospital-wide orientation, in-service, and continuing education programs directed toward the provision of quality care.

The role of the risk manager in quality assurance programs will either be direct or indirect. The risk manager may be an ex-officio member of some of the committees cited above and thus have a direct involvement. A more common approach to quality assurance participation is one of indirect involvement. Whether involvement is direct or indirect, the risk manager needs to be knowledgeable about all quality assurance activities and how they relate to the loss control program. In all instances specific problem situations should be given direct attention when intervention will reduce the hospital's liability exposure.

For example, in an incident involving a medication error an investigation conducted by the risk manager determined weaknesses in procedures of ordering, requisitioning, and distributing drugs. The situation was referred to an appropriate quality assurance committee for review. As a result, a new drug-handling system, involving physicians, nursing personnel, and pharmacists, was developed to alleviate this problem. Such an example demonstrates the close relationship that should and must exist between the quality assurance and risk management programs.

A significant amount of risk management can be conducted by having one committee know what the other committees are doing and by designating one person to synthesize all of the quality of care concerns expressed by the committees. In an increasing number of hospitals, the person designated to synthesize quality of care information is being referred to as a risk manager.[11]

Committee Functions

A brief explanation of committee functions could possibly be helpful in understanding the breadth of activities under a risk management program. It should be emphasized that the example just cited is not necessarily appropriate for every hospital. Other means may be just as effective or even more effective in fulfilling these functions. The point is that coordination of committee activities relating to the risk management function must exist.

The committees are generally charged with the responsibility of developing appropriate policies and procedures, as well as systems and methods to insure adherence to these policies and procedures. In general, each committee serves as a catalyst for activities relating to its purpose. Actions are subject to approval of the council and appropriate administrative levels within the organization, unless specifically delegated to committees.

The use of committees has been criticized by some management theorists as ineffective and a deterrent to organizational progress. This author once saw a sign on the wall of a hospital department that stated, "God so loved the world that He did not send a committee!" However, a committee structure in a staff activity such as risk management can prove to be very effective. It can be a means of insuring maximum and diversified involvement and interest throughout the organization. In a new program, these two ingredients are extremely important.

POLICIES AND PROCEDURES

Each hospital has its own method of developing a system for publishing operational policies and procedures. As previously noted, the establishment of such policies and procedures and putting them in written form is an important and necessary activity. Risk management without meaningful written guidelines will lack direction and consistency. Therefore, care in developing and publishing them must be exercised. As a general rule, hospitals should have four basic types of policies and/or procedures. These are:

1. *General Policy:* all hospital policies and procedures originate from the broad goals and objectives established by the governing body. It is the responsibility of the hospital administrator to translate these general concepts into administrative publications that (a) state the aims and principles governing action on particular functions and subjects, (b)

establish the organization responsible for carrying out such aims and acting on these principles, and (c) outline procedures necessary to implement aims.

2. *Standard Policy and Procedure (SPP):* all interorganizational policies, procedures, and instructions of a nonpersonnel nature are centralized in the Standard Policy and Procedure Manual.
3. *Personnel Policy and Procedure (PPP):* all interorganizational policies, procedures, and instructions relating to personnel and employment are centralized in the Personnel Policy and Procedure Manual.
4. *Departmental Policy and Procedure (DPP):* each department is responsible for developing, maintaining, and controlling a manual indicating intradepartmental policies, procedures, and instructions.

After recognizing the basic types of policies and procedures found in most hospitals, it is then necessary to formulate policies and procedures for the risk management program within each of these categories.

First, since all policy and procedures originate from the broad goals and objectives established by the governing body and translated into concepts by the hospital administration, it is important that a *general policy* statement be made at the governing and administrative levels to establish the impetus for this program. The following is an example:

_____ hospital is committed to providing a safe and secure environment within its facilities and grounds for all patients, visitors, employees, volunteers, and physicians. A formal program to prevent risks and harm to all persons involved in hospital services will be a part of the hospital's operations.

Second, policies and procedures should be developed by the risk manager specifically for the risk management program for an SPP manual. These will include the policies and procedures that have broad interorganization or interdepartmental connotations. Certain related SPPs will already exist, and these need only to be reviewed periodically to insure consistency with the risk management program. A few examples of SPP subjects relating directly or indirectly to the risk management program might include:

- patient admissions and identification
- incident/accident reporting
- infection surveillance
- lost and found
- drug management
- noise control

- patient valuables
- safety
- security
- smoking
- traffic control
- patient transfer and transportation
- visiting
- electrical safety
- environmental control

Third, because of the scope and significance of employee involvement in a human service organization such as a hospital, it is advantageous to develop a separate PPP manual. The PPP manual includes those interorganizational activities dealing primarily with personnel matters. Many of these also have risk management implications. Examples include:

- employee conduct
- traffic and parking regulations
- employee grievances/dissatisfactions
- material to and from hospital premises
- occupational injury and illness
- employee health
- safety responsibilities of employees
- key and card entry control
- employee deaths
- employee education
- personnel selection
- employee evaluation

Finally, SPPs and PPPs generally must be translated down to the departmental level. Here, many departments will have DPPs covering the same subjects. There will be other DPPs that are limited to only a single department. In such cases, these subjects will be covered in that department's DPP manual. The risk manager should develop guidelines for including loss-control matters in DPP manuals and review these inclusions to see that they are consistent with SPPs, as well as with operational aspects of the risk management program. A good example of this relationship between policies and procedures at the interorganizational, personnel, and intradepartmental levels is in the area of safety. General safety rules exist that are translated into personnel regulations and then defined specifically to satisfy each department's own safety needs. For example, in the SPP manual:

General Rules of Safety

- The purpose of the hospital's safety program is to provide a safe and healthful environment for the protection of all patients, visitors, employees, physicians, volunteers, and equipment and facilities.
- Accident prevention and efficient service go hand in hand. All hospital personnel share the responsibility for the safety, health, and well-being of patients, visitors, and staff. This responsibility can be met only by working together to promote a safe working environment.
- Safety rules apply to all personnel and all departments in the hospital. These, together with the specific departmental rules developed by the combined efforts of department heads and the Safety and Loss Control Council, should prove helpful in promoting safety consciousness and accident free operations.

Then a statement in the PPP manual:

Safety Responsibilities of Employees

- The hospital has a well-planned safety program. Copies of safety rules are filed in each department, and it is the responsibility of all employees to acquaint themselves with the program.
- Annual merit evaluations contain criteria related to safety performance of employees and will be used in determining merit increases in wages.

And finally in a housekeeping Department DPP manual:

Housekeeping Safety

- Mop up all spills and pick up hazardous objects.
- Consider yourself a member of the safety committee. Watch out for dangerous conditions.
- Do not handle trash with bare hands. Use gloves when using steel wool. Do not pick up broken glass; instead, sweep it up.
- Use the bottom of a wastebasket to push trash down in bigger containers.
- Do not place cleaning equipment on window sills when window is open. Injuries may be caused by falling objects.

One can easily see the close relationship that needs to exist between the different types and levels of policies and procedures to insure coordinated operational activity.

The need for good policies and procedures for the risk management program cannot be overstated. Policies and procedures are administrative tools that seek to insure consistency and conformity with organizational objectives.

It is one thing for a hospital to have proper policies and procedures; proving in a court of law that proper policies and procedures were followed is another matter. The hospital needs to examine its means of documenting exactly what care was provided, as well as all other operational activities governed by policies and procedures.[12]

THE TEAM APPROACH

The need to have involvement and commitment to the program at the governing and upper administrative levels has been mentioned previously. Also, the responsibilities of a key member of the risk management team, the risk manager, have been described in detail. But the governing body, the administrator, and the risk manager, though key members, are only a small part of the team that will be playing the serious game of loss prevention and control. In hospitals, whether they have 25 or 2500 beds, 1 or 500 doctors, or 15 or 1500 patients, a team approach to risk management is needed if the program is to reach its full potential. Who are the members of the team, and what part should each play in this program?

The risk management team includes the following: (1) governing body and administration, (2) risk manager, (3) department heads, (4) hospital employees (including volunteers), (5) the Safety and Loss-Control Council and related committees, (6) members of the medical staff, (7) hospital attorney, and (8) outside consultants. Certain functions and responsibilities are assigned to each team member, and each must fulfill these if the program, from an overall standpoint, is to be effective. The following team assignments are suggested:

1. Governing body and administration
   a. Define overall objectives and establish supportive atmosphere within the organization for the program
   b. Commit adequate resources of management, methods, manpower, material, and money to insure its success
   c. Require periodic progress reports and analyze the effectiveness of the program

2. Risk manager
   a. Provide management leadership and fulfill the appropriate staff role within the organization
   b. Assist other members of the team to fulfill their functions
3. Department heads
   a. Develop written departmental safety guidelines and include same in their departmental procedures manuals
   b. Consistently enforce all safety rules and regulations
   c. Be constantly alert for unsafe practices and unsafe conditions and be prepared to take appropriate action to correct any irregularities
   d. Investigate and complete reports on all incidents/accidents occurring in their area
   e. Instruct and train workers in safety, first aid, fire prevention, and disaster planning
   f. Provide and enforce the use of required safety devices and protective equipment
   g. Cooperate and assist with inspection tours of their departments
   h. Appoint employees to serve as members of the Safety and Loss Control Council and related committees
   i. Provide for preventive maintenance and repairs of departmental equipment
4. Employees
   a. Know and adhere to all safety and fire-prevention rules and regulations
   b. Report all unsafe practices and conditions to their supervisors
   c. Follow every precaution and safety rule to protect themselves, fellow employees, patients, and visitors
   d. Participate in fire and disaster drills as requested
   e. Report all injuries to their supervisors immediately
5. The Safety and Loss Control Council and other committees
   a. See that the hospital facility is maintained in a manner that protects the lives and assures the physical safety of its patients, its personnel, and its visitors
   b. See that the hospital is equipped and operated so as to sustain its safe, secure, and sanitary characteristics and to minimize all hazards
   c. Conduct periodic inspections of the hospital premises to detect unsafe and unhealthful conditions and practices and recommend appropriate corrective measures
   d. Analyze all accident and/or incident reports to determine causes and to suggest such remedial actions as may be appropriate to prevent recurrences

e. Compile and maintain an employee safety manual

f. Act in an advisory capacity to all department heads and supervisors to aid them in their safety responsibilities

g. Assist in periodic rehearsals of fire and disaster plans

h. Promote an ongoing educational program that will involve and inform all levels of hospital management and employees of their primary responsibility for the safety, health, and well-being of all patients, visitors, and hospital staff

*6. Members of the medical staff

*7. Hospital attorney

*8. Consultants and outside services

*Because of the uniqueness of these team members, a special section is being devoted to each.

MEDICAL STAFF PARTICIPATION

The hospital medical staff's traditional role within the hospital organization has been a somewhat isolated one when it comes to operational matters. The medical staff is self-governing and, to a large degree, self-policing (subject, of course, to the ultimate authority of the hospital governing body). Historically, this ultimate authority in many hospitals has been exercised in a rubber stamp manner. However, because hospital boards in recent years have been held liable not only for the actions of physicians but also for neglecting to exercise appropriate supervision over the quality of medical practice in the hospital, a new interdependent relationship is developing. Another factor causing this new comradeship is the fact that the greatest amount of malpractice litigation against physicians results from situations that occurred in the course of their hospital practice. This evolving relationship recognizes that both hospital and physician are in the same boat and, in general, are considered as one, particularly in relation to liability. Therefore, an unprecedented need exists for cooperation and teamwork between the hospital and its medical staff.

Medical Staff Committees

It goes without saying that physicians are the only ones qualified and licensed to practice medicine. To a large degree, they are also the only ones qualified to judge the professional aspects of medical practice in a hospital setting. For these reasons medical staff committees, collectively representing the hospital doctors, have special responsibilities as team members to assure quality medical practice. A structure to accomplish this exists in most hospitals, and it should be reinforced and supported by the governing body and administration. Committee activities seem to be a most effective means of implementing a program if properly structured and employed. Physician identification with risk management can easily be achieved through study of the existing medical staff committee structure.[13]

Some pertinent committee functions include:

- medical staff bylaws, rules, and regulations
- medical care evaluation and audit
- medical records and documentation
- medical diagnosis and treatment standards
- medical staff selection and privilege delineation
- medical staff education
- medical staff and departmental organization
- medical disaster (part of hospital disaster committee)
- patient care/professional liability

One means used, particularly in hospitals in Ohio, to prevent a breakdown in professional care, whether by the physician or hospital staff, is an audit of the quality of patient care by a Patient Care/Professional Liability Committee. The cardinal point in such a program is that the Patient Care/Professional Liability forum (a group composed of existing quality-evaluating professionals working in the hospital setting) works in conjunction with hospital monitoring of patient incidents and procedures. This arrangement allows regular review of incidents and analysis of incident patterns through a medical and nursing audit.[14]

A trend that was given impetus in recent years by the JCAH, American Medical Association, and American Hospital Association, has been to include nonphysicians on medical staff committees. This has allowed and encouraged communication with and education of all those involved.

Using the same logic, it is time to start involving physician members on nonmedical staff committees. In the area of risk management, it is particularly important to have physician members on the Safety and Loss Control Council and related committees. Many physicians will have neither the time nor the interest to serve on another committee or to be conscientious in offering professional input. In spite of this, with thoughtful selectivity and in consultation with the chief of staff, the right physician for each slot can be chosen. Hospitals, in general, should increase physician involvement in all of their operations.

Beyond actual formal involvement in such activities as committee work, the individual physician as a team member is of paramount importance. Mature, interested physicians can be valuable sources of constructive criticism and evaluation, with resulting improvements in hospital operations and, in the case of risk management, identification of problems.

Physician Profile

Because the medical staff is by nature *self-policing* (subject to the ultimate authority of the governing body), it has a responsibility to identify problem individuals and situations within its ranks. In addition to normal patient care evaluation activities conducted through committees, a medical staff is required to pass judgment on its individual members. Too often, the annual reappointment process results in a hurried, thoughtless recommendation for reappointment of all members with the same privileges, year after year.

In an effort to assist the medical staff and governing body in monitoring both staff privileges and annual reappointments, physician "profiles" are being developed in some hospitals.[15] In institutions with data-processing capacity, such a program is easily handled, but basic information can also be maintained manually for this purpose.

Some of the data that may be included in the profile follows:

- Physician's utilization of hospital facilities (including outpatient and emergency services)
- Physician's attendance of staff and committee meetings (including excused absences)
- Physician's continuing medical education credits earned
- Physician's participation in internal educational activities within the hospital (both as instructor and participant)
- Physician's specialty board eligibility or certification status
- Other basic information concerning such things as formal training, work experience, memberships on other staffs, liability insurance, and malpractice claim experience

If a medical staff is accurately to monitor and evaluate its members and then act appropriately in regard to them, such basic information needs to be available.

An Operational Barometer

Historically, physicians have not always approached problem situations in a rational manner. Despite this, their general attitudes can serve as a good barometer to measure the effectiveness of operational activities and give warning signals about areas of difficulty.

The hospital–physician relationship should be cordial enough for them to share information and problems, particularly in regard to risk situations. Anticipation of repercussions of incidents and accidents, when shared by the parties involved, usually results in a better approach to corrective action.

The risk manager should consider members of the medical staff as part of the risk management team and use them not only as resources but also as involved, contributing members. Because the physician and the hospital are so closely identified, the risk manager should consider the reduction of risk to individual members of the medical staff as much a part of the job as the prevention of loss to the hospital.

It is tempting to state at this point that doctors and hospitals will always cooperate and work together harmoniously in mutual interest and toward mutual objectives relative to the risk management program. Unfortunately, from a practical standpoint, this is just not always so. In problem situations, there is always a potential division between these parties when they find themselves as the accused parties or as codefendants in the same case. In this regard it should be emphasized that the hospital and doctor are generally looked upon as a single entity by those they serve. Therefore, a defense by one at the expense of the other party generally is the poorest approach to ultimate resolution. Conversely, the best approach to resolve successfully a potential risk situation will usually be a common and consistent one.

> Claims handling is a common ground that physicians and hospitals should reach immediately. The infighting that occurs after a suit is filed as each defendant named seeks to minimize or escape financial loss aids only the plaintiff. Mutual cooperation between physician and hospital is necessary if a suit is to be defended in a logical, efficient manner.[16]

HOSPITAL ATTORNEY'S ROLE

With the rapid growth of litigation against hospitals and the great increase in new laws and regulations, the role of the hospital attorney has evolved from a minor to a major one. The situation has changed so significantly in recent years that some hospitals have full-time lawyers on their staffs. Many have multiple attorneys to assist in specialty activities in such areas as labor, taxes, and trusts, as well as in the malpractice field.

The hospital attorney's primary responsibility is to represent the hospital in litigation proceedings. In addition the attorney may be designated as a person responsible for some of the operational activities. If a risk management program exists, there are many ways the hospital's legal counsel can assist other than in the courtroom.

Some of the specific functions fulfilled by the hospital attorney may include:

1. Advisor to the governing body relative to legal implications of bylaws, rules, regulations, policy establishment, and ultimate decisions made by the board; specifically, assists with legal documents, including resolutions, articles of incorporation, trust agreements, and contracts
2. Advisor to the medical staff relative to establishment and enforcement of bylaws, rules, and regulations; assists, when appropriate, medical staff committees dealing with medical evaluation and other related activities with legal implications
3. Assists directly, when needed, the hospital administrator in operational activities having legal implications
4. Advises designated members of the hospital team in operational matters having legal implications (Those designated may include assistant administrators, medical records administrator, director of nursing, admission director, personnel director, and risk manager.)

It is common today to have the attorney attend hospital board meetings. In some cases the attorney is an ex-officio member of that body. When multiple members of the administrative staff, in addition to the administrator, are given authority to make direct contact with the hospital attorney, it is important that this be spelled out in writing so that only legitimate use is made of this expensive resource.

The hospital attorney's relationship with the hospital carries with it the rights and privileges of any lawyer–client association. Information exchanged is privileged, and, therefore, this is an excellent way to store good, hard facts in all problem situations irrespective of their sometimes damaging nature.

In situations where liability insurance is carried by a hospital, the hospital attorney may not represent the insurance carrier when litigation occurs. In self-insurance situations the logical representative in courtroom proceedings is the hospital's general counsel unless specialty services are needed. An exception to this rule will occur when the hospital attorney does not have experience as a trial lawyer. With the inclusion in some states of binding arbitration, tort law changes, statutory pretrial review panels,[17] and other new methods in the handling of malpractice cases, legal specialists with expertise in these processes can prove most valuable.

In cases where potential liability occurs, many advantages exist in having an attorney represent the hospital who is familiar with and deeply committed to institutional activities. This is particularly true if the attorney becomes involved in situations soon after they are identified as serious potential risk incidents. Legal advice should be sought whenever potential liability is obvious or even considered a remote possibility in a situation or incident. An arrangement should be made with the hospital attorney to establish files on all serious risk incidents. Some institutions have a policy of establishing a legal file on all such situations. This can become very costly. Therefore, good judgment should be used in this regard.

The hospital attorney's role has changed and broadened dramatically in recent years. The hospital's legal counsel is no longer just a name on the list of resources, someone who draws a monthly retainer. Instead, the attorney is an active member of the operational team. The role will expand further with the establishment of such programs as self-insurance and risk management and with the increasing need to protect the institution's legal flank.

CONSULTANT AND OUTSIDE SERVICES

In risk management, as in other programs, consultants or outside services serve two basic purposes; they provide necessary expertise, which is not available within the organization, and/or they serve to enhance and improve existing activities necessary for an effective program. The use of outsiders on the hospital team is an established practice that has been in existence for many years. Clinical services (e.g., pathology, radiology, anesthesiology, pharmacy) and general services (e.g., dietary, housekeeping, laundry, maintenance) are provided in many hospitals on contractual bases with outsiders.

When selecting a consultant or consultant firm to assist in a risk management program, basic principles should be followed, as in any other contract for service. A judicious analysis and projection of the needs of a hospital is the starting point for administrators or their designates who are considering the utilization of outside services. When the decision for contracting is made, five major steps should be taken before a contract is signed. These steps are:

1. Prepare specifications for the service that incorporates everything that is expected of the consultant.
2. Request bids for the service from only reputable consultants or firms.
3. Investigate all bidders who respond with quotations to make certain they can fulfill their promise.
4. Evaluate the quality of service as well as its price, and then award the contract to the lowest bidder when quality is equal.
5. Prepare a contract that clearly enumerates your requirements, and make sure it is signed by a person in authority in the consultant firm.

Hospital administrators should be aware of the principal mechanics, and advantages, and disadvantages inherent in the use of consultant services in their hospitals, and their decision to purchase such services should be as objective as possible. There is value in reviewing the experiences of other hospitals who use such services before signing any contract. Ultimately, all contractual arrangements for consultant services should be weighed individually, and a final decision should be based on the merits and demerits of each service.[18]

In the area of risk management, certain outside consultant services have been used effectively. Some of the areas in which consultants have been used are:

1. General risk management and loss prevention
2. Risk analysis and evaluation
3. Safety and security programs
4. Self-insurance functions
   a. Actuarial services
   b. Claims surveillance and adjustment
   c. Trust establishment and management

As risk management programs become more popular and recognized as a viable, feasible activity, consultant services in other risk-related areas will probably come into existence and serve a useful purpose. It should be noted that in institutions that have outside insurance programs, the insurance carriers or underwriters serve as consultants to the organizations for many of these services.

A statement by Frank J. Dawson about contracting for outside services puts into words the philosophy that should be uppermost in the mind of the administrator when selecting this course of action.

> It has been said that a hospital is judged not by its rules but by the exceptions to those rules that it is able to render gracefully. A [consultant] service which directly or indirectly affects the patient is more than just an ordinary purchase by the hospital and should be so assessed by the administrator. The sole purpose of [such a] service, it would seem, is to augment the institution's ability to provide better patient care. The outside arrangement for inside service must render itself personable and flexible in the hands of administration.[19]

THE RISK MANAGEMENT OFFICE

The office is the home base for many organizational functions and generally serves as an action center. Here, the term *risk management office* is used generically to describe the center of specific day-to-day activities involved in a risk management program. This office may be located as an extension of an existing department or it may be autonomous with full departmental status. As previously mentioned, the organizational setting of the program, just as the organizational status of the risk manager, are determinations that must be made by individual hospitals.

In the AHA manual, *Controlling Hospital Liability: A Systems Approach,* the concept of a hospital liability control center is introduced. In regard to this concept, a premise is made

> ... that the hospital already possesses information critical to averting claims or reducing financial severity ... most of this information lies in file drawers and memories until a claim is filed against the hospital. Then, the bits and pieces of data unfold like a set of clues in a Sherlock Holmes story. The liability control system starts its detective work on these clues before or immediately after the claim is filed. The system provides a pathway through the volumes of information developed in the hospital, identifies clues that portend a possible claim, and mobilizes appropriate remedial action. Various existing hospital systems feed information into the liability control center.[20]

Under this concept, the risk management office is the logical liability control center and the risk manager is the logical liability control administrator. A central clearinghouse for information is essential, although other functions are equally important to the success of the risk management program. Some of the basic functions of the office should include:

- receiving, logging, and maintaining incident/accident reports and support information
- maintaining pertinent records and minutes of related committee activities
- preparing appropriate statistical analyses and reviews from gathered information
- coordinating the activities of related committees
- initiating immediate follow-up to risk problem situations
- coordinating and supplementing risk prevention and corrective activities throughout the organization
- performing other related activities as the need arises

The risk management office should not be considered just a receiver of information. A more important function is to initiate and support appropriate action directed toward prevention and correction of risk situations. Many times, after an incident or bad outcome, a simple visit by a representative of the hospital to the patient or patient's family could soothe tempers and avoid misinformation. In this way, a claim against the hospital might be averted.[21] A responsive risk management office should give the impetus for such activities. The risk management office is at the core of the liability control system. This home base for the risk management program, wherever it is located organizationally, receives and dispenses information resulting in active processes directed toward managing the hospital's risks.

CONCLUSION

If ten different hospitals were to be visited, one would discover ten distinctly different organizations. Although similarities would exist, the many differences among them would also become apparent. The organizations would be different because the needs of each would be dissimilar; the community that each served would be unique; the available personnel, material, and financial resources would be varied; the age and condition of each facility would not be the same; the administrative leadership styles practiced would be different; and so on.

The same phenomenon also holds true in individual institutional activities. In establishing an organizational framework for any activity, it is extremely important that the structure be designed so it will support and not hinder the activity. Remember that the purpose of organizational development is to facilitate accomplishment of institutional goals.

In organizing a program such as risk management, the uniqueness of the hospital needs to be given prime consideration. For this reason it is important that each hospital that is evaluating the inclusion of risk management first survey its needs in regard to loss control and liability prevention. It is fine to follow certain guidelines and principles; of equal importance is the desirability that risk management activities be tailor-made to fit institutional requirements.

As is true in most institutional functions, risk management is created neither by a magic formula nor a set recipe. Its organizational character will develop differently in each hospital. Variations in the organizational framework are of minor significance, as long as the purposes of risk management programs are fulfilled. Because of this, a sense of flexibility and adaptability should definitely accompany efforts to establish such a function within the organization.

This chapter has cited many principles and examples in regard to program organization. The principles may serve as helpful guidelines, but each example should be treated as only one of many different approaches which may be followed in the erection of a risk management organizational structure.

RISK MANAGEMENT ORGANIZATION CHECKLIST

___ Are existing activities in place which will provide necessary support of a risk management program?

___ Is the risk management function located organizationally in a *staff* department or division?

___ Have necessary management, manpower, methods, materials, and money been committed to the program?

Risk manager

___ Has a risk manager been designated?

___ Does the risk manager have strengths in organizational developments, creativeness, interpersonal relations, and persuasive ability?

___ Is the title *risk manager* or other descriptive designation used to establish program identity?

___ Has a job description for the risk manager been developed?

Organizational structure

___ Are related committees currently functioning in such areas as safety, environment control, disaster, and education?

___ Are the activities of these committees formally coordinated and integrated to improve communication and effectiveness?

___ Does an overall risk management coordinating committee exist in some form?

___ Does the risk management program involve multiple disciplines, as well as administrative, supervisory, and nonsupervisory levels?

Policies and procedures

___ Is there a general policy established by the governing body relative to risk management or loss prevention?

___ Does standard policy and procedure (SPP) include interorganizational policies and procedures related to risk management?

___ Does personnel policy and procedure (PPP) include risk management related activities?

___ Does departmental policy and procedure (DPP) include each department's activities related to risk management?

The team

___ Does a team approach philosophy exist in the organization?

___ Do members of the hospital organization consider themselves involved and responsible in risk management?

___ Are team assignments formalized for the governing body, administration, risk manager, department heads, employees, committees, medical staff, hospital attorney, and consultants?

Medical staff

___ Is the working relationship with the medical staff effective as it relates to risk management and problem solving?

___ Are pertinent medical staff committees functioning effectively to assure quality medical care in the hospital?

___ Is there nonphysician involvement in medical staff committees and physician involvement in risk management committees?

Hospital attorney

___ Does the hospital have a general counsel?

___ Is the role of the hospital attorney defined?

___ Is the attorney involved in the risk management program?

Consultants

___ Are consultants or outside contracts used to enhance the risk management program?

___ Are there weaknesses in the program that could be improved with the use of consultants with special expertise?

___ Were good principles followed in selecting consultants?

Note: This checklist is not meant to be all inclusive nor does it require absolute adherence. Its purpose is to stimulate thought and redirect attitudes toward the establishment of a risk management program.

NOTES

1. G. Newman, "Basic Elements of a Loss Control Program," *Hospital Progress,* November 1974, p. 46.

2. Y. Bryant and A. Korsak, "Who is the Risk Manager, and What Does He Do?" *Hospitals, JAHA,* January 16, 1978, p. 42.

3. J. Schmitt, "Risk Management Justification: Cost/Benefit Considerations," *Risk Management,* July 1977, p. 40.

4. C. Lenhard, "Building a Result-Oriented Control Program," *Risk Management,* July 1977, p. 18.

5. Bryant and Korsak, p. 42.

6. T. Dankmyer and J. Groves, "Taking Steps for Safety's Sake," *Hospitals, JAHA,* May 16, 1977, p. 60.

7. T. Chittenden, "Role of Physicians in Malpractice Needs Careful Exploration," *Hospitals, JAHA,* May 16, 1977, p. 55.

8. Newman, p. 49.

9. *Quality Assurance Program for Medical Care in the Hospital* (Chicago, Ill.: American Hospital Association, 1972), Sec. 2, p. 1.

10. "Quality Assurance and Risk Management Programs" (Phoenix, Ariz.: Samaritan Health Service, 1976), unpublished, p. 4.

11. M. Grayson, "Risk Management: New Focus for Traditional Functions," *The Hospital Medical Staff,* May 1978, p. 14.

12. *Controlling Hospital Liability: A Systems Approach,* developed and written by the Maryland Hospital Education Institute (Chicago, Ill.: American Hospital Association, 1976), p. 18.

13. M. Grayson, p. 14.

14. Lenhard, p. 8.

15. "Quality Assurance and Risk Management Programs," p. 14.

16. C. Davis, "Why Aggrieved Patients Sue Multiple Defendants," *The Hospital Medical Staff,* March 1978, p. 16.

17. *Legal Topics Relating to Medical Malpractice* (Washington, D.C.: U.S. Department of Health, Education, and Welfare Public Health Service, 1977), p. 2.

18. B. Brown, "Contract Services: Outsiders on the Hospital Team," *Hospital Topics,* August 1965, p. 64.

19. F. Dawson, "Purchasing: Outside Contracts for Inside Services," *Hospitals, JAHA,* July 1, 1961, p. 51.

20. *Controlling Hospital Liability,* pp. 2–3.

21. Ibid.

Chapter 4

Handling Potential Liability Problems

A totally safe environment is a place where risks do not exist. The word *safe* is defined as free from risk or harm. But in real life, absolute safety is a myth.[1] It goes without saying that all hospitals desire to function perfectly and be devoid of problems. In recognizing this impossibility, the realist will plan means of handling any problems that arise. In spite of all efforts to prevent and correct risk situations, serious incidents or accidents will occur periodically. In these cases, the risk management program can prove its worth if efforts of the program result in elimination or reduction of claim adjustments or settlements. Many times the initial handling of such situations immediately after they occur is critical in regard to the ultimate outcome in terms of liability cost.

In respect to the handling of potential liability problems, there are several general steps that should be followed as a part of the risk management program. First, and most obvious, is the identification of problem situations through appropriate incident/accident reports or other means. Second, a process of screening and determining the seriousness of each problem must be accomplished. Third, review, analysis, and resolution of the individual problem situations as well as corrective action relative to trends and patterns are necessary. Fourth, a follow-up system to correct or eliminate as much as possible the negative results of the incident/accident must be established. Fifth and final, when all else fails and a lawsuit is imminent, a logical system of litigation preparation must be used.

The flow of data and facts through this five-step process is crucial because this information will be used extensively in making decisions and in efforts to resolve risk situations. Figure 4-1 illustrates the flow process in the handling of potential liability problems. It should be noted when reviewing this illustration that resolution of problems can occur at any point along the route. Hopefully, many are resolved early. A few, though, will follow the entire process and be ultimately settled in a court of law.

Figure 4-1 Flow Process in Handling Potential Liability Problems

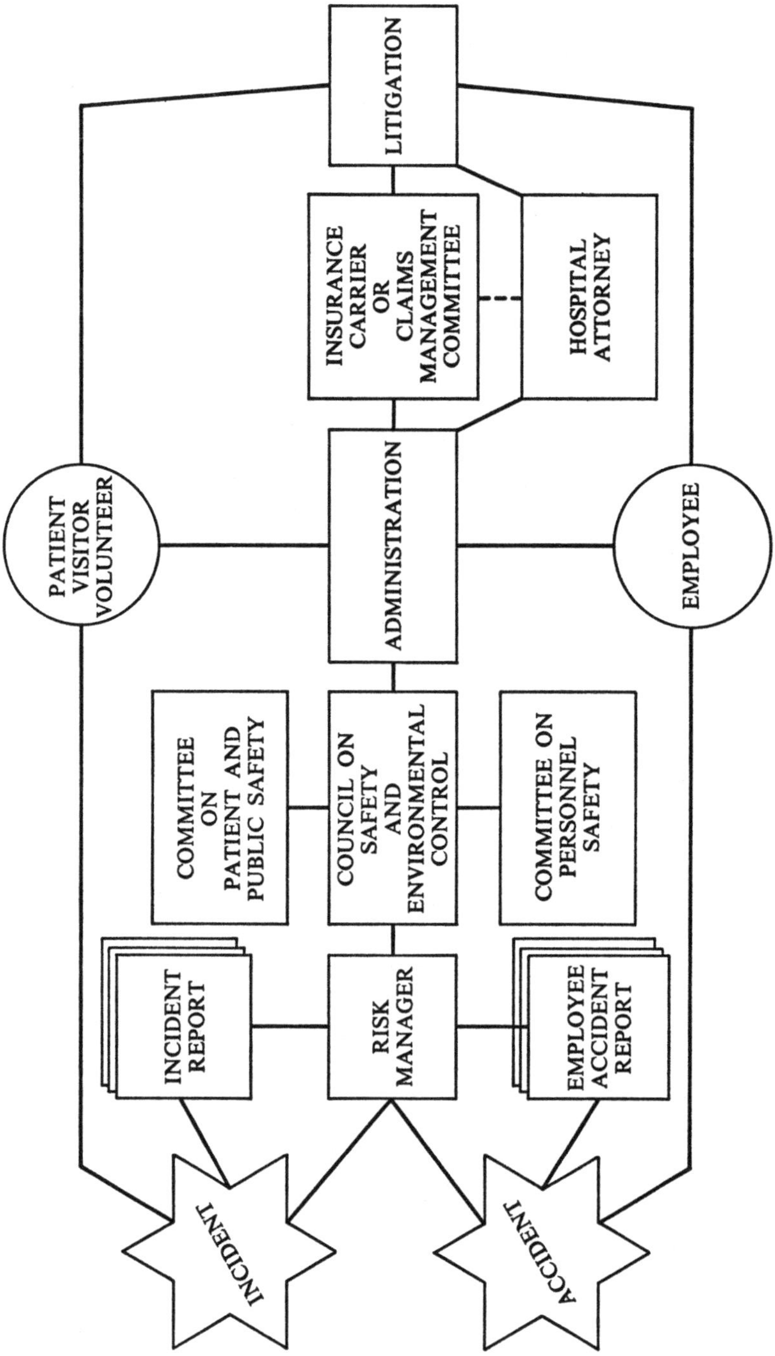

In discussing the handling of problem situations, one must remember that the actual performance of certain functions will vary depending on the hospital's organizational setup. Some of the influencing factors include:

- whether the hospital is externally insured or self-insured
- how comprehensive the risk management program is
- whether outside consultants are retained to assist in some of the functions
- how large and competent the administrative staff is
- other idiosyncrasies and characteristics of the organization

To illustrate how one of these factors may influence handling of problem situations, consider a hospital that has changed from a commercial to a self-insurance program. Prior to the change, the insurance carrier through its claims adjustment department probably handled much of the investigative work, made contact with those involved, and sought settlement of the issue. After the self-insurance program has been established, the same functions must occur; however, the institution finds that it must carry out these activities internally through its own risk management program. Though certain necessary steps must be taken, who actually is responsible for each step will vary, depending on factors such as those listed above.

Even though the uniqueness of individual hospitals may influence the handling of specific duties involved in problem solving, the basic activities of (1) identification, (2) centralizing information, (3) screening, (4) review, analysis and resolution, follow-up, and (5) litigation (if necessary) should be formalized in the risk management process.

IDENTIFICATION OF PROBLEMS

In most hospitals incident reports are the primary tools used in identifying risk situations that have occurred. However, incident reports alone are not adequate. There may be times when such a report is not completed for one reason or another, yet a problem is subsequently discovered and needs handling. Therefore, other sources of information should be recognized, including the following:

- incidents reported verbally by physicians and employees
- patient complaints to employees, administration, and the business office
- patient ombudsman findings
- letters from attorneys about injuries or other cases of patient dissatisfaction

- malpractice claims
- summaries of past claims experience or the experience of other hospitals
- inspections of the physical plant and audits of policies and procedures, such as relevant positions on the JCAH accreditation report
- the experience of employees and physicians
- findings of the medical audit or other quality assurance committees[2]

Regardless of the identification source of problem situations, as complete documentation as possible should be obtained. Even the use of incident reports prepared retrospectively can be helpful.

Investigation is an important part of problem identification. Investigative techniques cited in Chapter 2 can prove most helpful in this process. The real problem is not always obvious; those involved will view a problem situation from diverse perspectives and at times will perceive the cause and effect differently.

Incidents and Accidents

Some institutions may wish to classify all unusual happenings as incidents. However, because of the growing implications and complexities related to employee safety and security, a logical distinction can be made between a general incident involving patients, visitors, or volunteers and personnel accidents resulting in harm to employees. For purposes of definition, then, an *incident* means a risk situation that involves patients and the public in general; an *accident* is defined as one that involves employees.[3]

Because of the variations in necessary data and information, it is recommended that different report forms be designed for incidents and for accidents. A unique format for each will allow the reports to fulfill their respective purposes and will also provide adequate space for all pertinent information.

Basic information on the incident report (Exhibit 4-1) should consist of:

1. Personal data on patient, visitor, or volunteer for identification purposes
2. Designation of category of individual(s) involved in incident and information related to condition(s)
3. Description of incident from those involved and related supporting data
4. Physician's statement and analysis

Exhibit 4-1 Incident Report

			For Addressograph
Person involved: (Last name)	(First name)	(Middle initial)	Date of report
Age:	Male ( )		Female ( )

	Room no.	State cause for hospitalization
Patient ( )	Patient's condition before incident	
	Normal ( ) Senile ( ) Disoriented ( ) Sedated ( ) Other ( )	
	Were bed rails present Yes ( ) No ( ) Up ( ) Down ( )	Height of bed Up ( ) Down ( )
Visitor ( )	Home address	Home phone
Other ( )	Occupation and place of employment	
	Reason for presence at hospital	

CONFIDENTIAL REPORT OF INCIDENT

Exact location of incident	Date of incident	Time of incident a.m. ( ) p.m. ( )

Employee's account of incident (Describe exactly what happened)

_____

_____

_____

Physical evidence retained (supplies, instruments, etc.)

Statements made by person involved (If possible indicate quotes, note time, and to whom)

_____

_____

_____

Witnesses or persons familiar with incident

Name_____ Address_____

Name_____ Address_____

Name_____ Address_____

Physician notified: Yes ( ) No ( )	Time: a.m. ( ) p.m. ( )	Name of physician
Was person seen by physician Yes ( ) No ( )	Time: a.m. ( ) p.m. ( )	Where

Physician's statement:

Additional comments:

_____

Source: Adaptation of form used by Kennestone Hospital, Marietta, Georgia, 1978.

Exhibit 4-2 Accident Report

EMPLOYEE	Name: (Last) (First) (Middle Initial)	Department:
INJURED	Job Title: Status Full time ( ) Part time ( )	Hours per pay period

	Date of accident	Time of accident (a.m.) (p.m.)	Date accident reported by employee
	Date lost time began	Time Lost time began (a.m.) (p.m.)	Employee paid for day of accident Yes ( ) No ( )
DETAILS	To whom accident reported	Name of supervisor
OF	Was accident caused by failure to:	Use safety equipment Observe safety Yes ( ) No ( ) rules Yes ( ) No ( )
ACCIDENT	Describe how accident occurred and why (Use back if necessary)
	_____
	_____
	_____
	Name of instrument causing accident, if any	Location of accident
	Was accident due to: Employee's action ( ) Action of others ( ) Equipment failure ( )
	Name and address of witness:
	Nature and location of injury (Right or left side, hand or knee, etc.)
	Has injured returned to work Yes ( ) No ( )	If returned, indicate date and time
	Signature and title of person preparing report	Date

	Emergency physician's name:	Date and time seen: (a.m.) (p.m.)	Where examined
EMERGENCY	Emergency physician's statement (Use back if necessary)
MEDICAL	_____
INFORMATION	_____
	_____
	Estimated return to work date	Private physician name, if referred

PERSONNEL	Social security number	Address of employee
DEPARTMENT	Employment date	Marital Status: Single ( ) Married ( ) Divorced ( ) Widowed ( ) Separated ( )
USE ONLY	Sex Male ( ) Female ( )	Birthdate	Home telephone	Rate of pay
	Actual return to work date	Medical charges
	Disposition

Source: Adaptation of form used by Kennestone Hospital, Marietta, Georgia, 1978.

The information contained in the accident report (Exhibit 4-2) should consist of:

1. Employee identification data
2. Details of the accident
3. Emergency medical information
4. Pertinent personnel information

The use of incident/accident reports should be required and promoted for problem identification purposes. Some may feel that the documentation of problem situations will inflict criticism upon those responsible. This attitude should be emphatically discouraged. Actually, the completion of incident/accident reports demonstrates the conscientiousness and concern of those involved. These reports are positive and not negative tools, and the old human-nature deterrents of "not getting involved" and "being defensive" should be eliminated.

In the past, the incident/accident report form was too often used solely to help establish the hospital's defense in a lawsuit resulting from a claim. If used properly, this form can help prevent many claims from being filed in the first place. All appropriate hospital staff should be instructed in the use of the form and encouraged to file their reports immediately after incidents have taken place. For safety's sake, even seemingly inconsequential incidents should be reported.[4] It is important to remember that an environment in which reprisals are allowed for reporting errors is counterproductive.[5]

The method for handling an incident should be a part of the standard policy and procedure (SPP) manual of the hospital. An example of such an SPP follows.

SPP: General Incidents

Purpose
To define general incidents and the responsibilities associated with reporting, investigating, and handling them as effectively as possible.
Policy
To promptly and accurately document and investigate cases involving patients, visitors, and volunteers. To provide immediate medical assistance when necessary to those injured or ill as a result of the incident.
General Information
  1. An incident is any happening that is not consistent with the routine operation of the hospital or the routine care of a particular patient. It may be an accident or a situation that results in an accident.
  2. An incident report must be completed in duplicate for all incidents involving patients, visitors, or volunteers within the

hospital or hospital property. Department heads or supervisors are responsible for completing incident reports for all situations occurring within their area of responsibility. Incidents occurring outside the hospital and those occurring on hospital property and undefined areas, such as corridors, stairways, and elevators, should be reported by any employee witnessing the happening or by the attending emergency services staff if the victim is brought there for treatment.

3. It is important that this report be completed immediately, describing the details of the incident as accurately as possible. The original copy should be routed to the risk management office (or office responsible for this function) and the copy sent to the appropriate division in which the incident occurred for review and follow-up investigation as required.

4. Employees should make no statements to patients or visitors about the ultimate outcome or disposition of an incident. Only after a complete investigation of all facts will the hospital be able to make any determination of appropriate action. Specific inquiries may be referred to the risk manager or responsible division head.

5. The risk management office will insure that all incident reports are maintained and routinely reported to the Patient and Public Safety Committee for their review and evaluation in accordance with committee procedures.

6. It is the policy of the hospital to waive hospital charges for routine emergency medical examinations in the emergency services department following incidents involving any visitor to the hospital or on hospital property. The provision of these emergency services is performed as a matter of courtesy to the person involved.

Responsibility and Authority

1. Department head or supervisor shall:

   a. When advised of an incident involving a patient, visitor, or volunteer, complete an incident report and insure that the injured/ill person receives prompt medical attention.

   b. Distribute the incident report as indicated in General Information: Item 3.

   c. Consult with the risk manager and, if determined appropriate, investigate the scene of the incident to determine the nature and/or existence of safety hazards; request corrective action as required. Consult with other departments as necessary in this regard.

2. Risk Manager (or designated department) shall:

a. Upon receipt of an incident report, insure that the details are recorded properly and assist in investigation of the incident.

b. Working with the patient accounts department, see that charges for immediate medical attention are waived as a courtesy.

c. Notify the appropriate administration representatives and the hospital's insurance carrier and/or individual (consultant) handling claims surveillance/adjustments.

d. Maintain records and make reports on all incidents in accordance with the activities of the Patient and Public Safety Committee.

The method for handling an employee accident resulting in occupational injury or illness should be included in the Personnel Policy and Procedure (PPP) manual. An example of this PPP is as follows:

PPP: Occupational Injury or Illness

Purpose

To promote a safe environment for all hospital personnel by properly handling, investigating, and medically treating all employee injuries or illnesses occurring while performing regularly assigned work duties for the hospital.

Policy

To promptly and accurately document and investigate such cases to comply with the Occupational Safety and Health Act and Workmen's Compensation Law.

General Information

1. An occupational injury is any injury that results from a work accident or from exposure to hazards in the work environment. An occupational illness is any abnormal condition or disorder, other than one resulting from an occupational injury, caused by exposure to environmental factors associated with employment.

2. Any injury or illness sustained in the performance of work should be reported promptly to the employee's supervisor or department head, who is responsible for completing an employee accident report in duplicate. If the injury requires no medical attention, the report is completed and the original copy is forwarded to the risk management office (or department respon-

sible for this function) for processing. The duplicate copy is forwarded to the affected division head and returned to the department for retention in departmental records. When medical attention is necessary and the original accident form has been completed by the emergency services department, the form is forwarded to the risk management department for processing. The report will be coordinated with the personnel department.

3. Minor emergency services department charges and related minor hospital pharmacy expenses for treatment of an occupational injury that results in a disability of seven (7) days or less will normally be waived. Major medical expenses incurred by referral to a private physician or compensation expenses in an occupational disability of eight days or more will be covered by the hospital's workmen's compensation insurance carrier.

4. All full- and part-time employees of the hospital are covered by workmen's compensation provisions of the laws of the state.

Responsibility and Authority

1. Employee incurring occupational injury or illness should:

a. Notify immediate supervisor and report to the emergency services department for treatment. When the injury is serious, proceed directly for medical treatment even if the supervisor is unavailable for notification.

b. If the injury results in a disability of eight (8) or more days, obtain a physician's written statement indicating a possible time of work resumption.

2. Department heads or supervisors shall:

a. When advised of an occupational injury or illness, complete an employee accident report and assure that employee receives prompt medical attention. In serious injuries assure that medical treatment is provided expeditiously.

b. Distribute the accident report as indicated in General Information: Item 2.

c. Investigate the scene of the accident, injury, or illness to determine the nature and/or existence of safety hazards and request corrective action as required. Consult with risk manager and/or personnel director.

d. Advise employee of policies related to occupational injury or illness.

3. Emergency Services or Employee Health Department shall:

a. Promptly treat an employee who incurs injury or illness on hospital premises.

b. Complete physician's statement portion of accident report and return to risk management office.

c. Refer injured employee to hospital pharmacy when prescription drugs are required.

4. Risk Management or Personnel Department shall:

a. Upon receipt of accident report, assure that details are recorded according to Occupational Safety and Health Act and Workmen's Compensation laws.

b. Waive minor emergency services department treatment expenses for occupational injuries that result in disability of seven (7) days or less.

c. Notify workmen's compensation carrier of injury/illness and developments as they occur.

d. Maintain records and make reports on all occupational injuries or illnesses in accordance with the hospital's Employee Safety Committee procedures, the Occupational Safety and Health Act, and Workmen's Compensation laws.

CENTRALIZATION OF INFORMATION

A systematic method of centrally recording incidents and accidents is essential to the program. Whenever an incident that has potential liability occurs, a central file with documentation must be established.[6] This information located in a liability control center will provide immediate access for subsequent activities involved in the handling of risk situations.[7] The risk manager will administer the liability control center, which will serve as a clearinghouse for all pertinent information dealing with potential risk problems. In addition to incident/accident reports, other materials, such as related committee minutes, investigative reports, support documents, and other appropriate information, will be maintained in this center.

For incident reports (involving patients, visitors, volunteers, etc.), a basic logging system can be used. Basic information in the log should include:

- log number
- identification code number
- age
- date
- time
- unit
- incident description

In the case of accident reports (involving employees), a similar log sheet may be used. In these cases, additional reports, including OSHA No. 200,

Log of Occupational Injuries and Illness, must be maintained. This form includes:

- case or file number
- date
- employee information
- description of injury or illness
- extent of and outcome of cases[8]

Where possible, the identification of patients, visitors, employees, and others involved in incident/accidents should be coded rather than named. This assists in maintaining confidentiality as well as in promoting objective and consistent handling of the situations.

Incident reports should not be placed on the medical chart, and there should be no notation that an incident report has been filled out. It is not necessary to indict yourself. Chart only *what* has happened, not *why*. Copies going to the hospital attorney should contain the patient's name. Other copies and logged information should be coded.

SCREENING PROCESS

After receiving an incident or accident report and completing an investigation of the situation, the risk manager should determine whether the problem has a major or minor potential for liability. Some institutions may not wish to make a distinction in this regard. However, if the use of incident and accident reports is encouraged or required for all unusual happenings, a great number of these reports will probably be generated. Therefore, there seems to be some advantage in making this distinction, so that minor incident/accidents can be handled routinely and major ones can be given special attention. Where the difference is indistinguishable, the risk manager should probably rate an incident/accident as major to be safe. To utilize limited resources most effectively, the hospital should identify the most likely areas or procedures that expose the hospital to the filing of claims. A liability control approach should concentrate first on these high-risk priorities.[9] Effective risk managers cannot have paranoid tendencies; they must be able to separate real from imaginary risks. A risk manager who cries wolf too often will not be believed when the real potential disaster is uncovered.[10]

All minor and major incident/accident reports will be routed to the appropriate committees (incidents to the Patient and Public Safety Committee and accidents to the Personnel Safety Committee) for routine review and recommendations. Additionally, major ones will be reviewed immediately with the appropriate administrative representative (administrator, associate administrator, or assistant administrator) and the medical representative (member of safety committee, chairman of appropriate medical service, or attending physician), if the incident has medical care implications. These reports along with support information will also be sent immediately to the hospital attorney who will establish an active file on the incident. Those with possible malpractice implications should be referred immediately to the hospital legal counsel.[11]

A major part of the screening process is the determination of the attitudes of individuals and/or families who have suffered as the result of an incident/accident. This is particularly important in determining the significance of the situation. At times, serious situations may not be given enough attention by those involved, while minor ones are often blown up out of proportion and made to seem like major ones. The attitude of those involved is certainly not the only criterion one may use to make the classification but it is one of the main factors.

In regard to handling problems, this question often is asked, "Who is the best institutional representative to make contact and discuss the situation with the victim or victims of an accident (or incident)?" There is no simple answer to this question. A general answer is, "The person who can best relate to or develop a good rapport with those involved and, at the same time, look out for the interests of the hospital." Depending on the circumstances, this may be the attending physician, the head nurse on the unit, the director of nursing, a department head, an administrative representative, or the risk manager. One aspect of this question that is often overlooked is the desirability of deferred decisions. A person on a lower echelon can gracefully delay by passing the buck, whereas top-echelon officials may feel more pressured to make spur-of-the-moment decisions. Again, circumstances of the situation influence this determination. Judgment with finesse is the key to this selection. Positive and active thought should be given to this decision because it may be a determining factor in the ultimate resolution of the problem.

Many approaches may be used in the initial as well as subsequent contacts of a hospital representative with involved individuals. Certain guidelines may prove helpful in this difficult but necessary duty.

1. Remember that victims of an incident or accident will probably be upset and irritated and may be aggressive, accusing, and belligerent. Because of this, a special need exists to be calm, understanding, and concerned.
2. Mainly listen. They may need to let off steam, and you do not want to say anything that will further aggravate the situation.
3. Make notes. This assists documentation as well as letting complainants know you are listening and are serious in your concern.

4. Attempt to reassure without making any inappropriate commitments. Indicate that a full investigation will be held and promise follow-up.
5. Expressing personal interest or experience may also be helpful. (Use your best judgment in this regard.)
6. A good way to close the conversation is to indicate that the hospital is here to help people, and the last thing one would desire is that a person might be injured or harmed in an incident/accident. An honest, sincere, and sympathetic spirit should be maintained throughout the contact.

REVIEW, ANALYSIS, AND RESOLUTION

As a part of the review and analysis process, forms in addition to the basic incident/accident reports may be used and can prove valuable. These usually serve the purpose of reminding those investigating, reviewing, and analyzing situations of pertinent questions that need to be answered or steps that need to be taken. A critical incident/accident investigation form (Exhibit 4-3) and a medication and treatment errors and omissions form (Exhibit 4-4) are examples of these special purpose tools.

After the basic facts are accumulated, support information is obtained, and input from all involved is received, review and analysis leading to recommendations and decisions must occur. There are basically two types of review and analysis processes. The first deals with the individual situation and its resolution. The second involves general trends that may be discovered when reviewing all incidents/accidents and determining appropriate steps that need to be taken to reverse these trends.

Individual Problems

In regard to individual situations, one will ask, "How should this specific problem involving an incident/accident be resolved?" From the hospital's standpoint, there are basically four choices available to those making decisions. The availability of facts and the use of judgment will determine the selection. These choices are:

1. *Accept no responsibility.* This decision is usually made when the facts indicate no negligence or improper actions on the part of the hospital or its staff (or, in the case of employees, where workmen's compensation laws do not apply). This course of action may also be selected if the attitude of those involved is positive and no demand has been made that the institution accept responsibility.
2. *Accept limited responsibility.* Many times a gesture or expression of good will in the form of accepting limited responsibility is enough to resolve the issue and satisfy those involved. An example of this course is

Exhibit 4-3 Critical Incident Investigation Form

DATE: _____

TIME: _____

PATIENT'S NAME: _____

COMPLAINANT'S NAME: _____

RELATIONSHIP TO PATIENT: _____

_____

NATURE OF COMPLAINT (Please include full description): _____

_____

_____

_____

_____

IMMEDIATE ACTION: _____

_____

_____

_____

FOLLOWUP ACTION: _____

_____

_____

_____

ASSESSMENT AND RECOMMENDATION: _____

_____

_____

_____

_____
(Signature)

_____
(Title)

Source: Adaptation of form used by Kennestone Hospital, Marietta, Georgia, 1978.

Exhibit 4-4 Medication and Treatment Errors and Omissions

MEDICATION AND TREATMENT ERRORS AND OMISSIONS

Date of discovery of error_____
Name of physician notified_____
   Date and time_____
   Notified by whom_____
Name of supervisor (if notified)_____
Other persons notified_____   (Use patient addressograph)

Name of person(s) who made error_____
   ( ) Unit_____ ( ) Full time   ( ) Part time   ( ) R.N.   ( ) L.P.N.
   ( ) Student (Specify school)_____
Date and time of error _____
Diagnosis of patient_____
List medicine or medicines involved_____
Brief description of error (How discovered and effect on patient - sequence of events and other
   persons involved)_____
_____
_____
_____
_____

CAUSE(S) OF ERROR(S). CHECK BELOW.

1. Failure to follow procedure:
   ( ) a. Identification of patient.
   ( ) b. Didn't check medicine label with kardex.
   ( ) c. Didn't check route of administration.
   ( ) d. Didn't wait until patient took medicine.
   ( ) e. Didn't chart medication immediately.
   ( ) f. Not charted correctly.
   ( ) g. Not charted promptly.

2. Communication failure
   ( ) a. Not written correctly.
   ( ) b. Not read correctly.
   ( ) c. Not heard correctly.
   ( ) d. T.L. was not notified of "STAT" medication.
   ( ) e. "STAT" order was not sent to pharmacy.
   ( ) f. "STAT" order was not received from pharmacy.

3. ( ) Wrong calculation

4. ( ) Lack of concentration

5. ( ) Drug not available on unit

6. ( ) Other _____

TO BE COMPLETED BY HEAD NURSE,
SUPERVISOR, OR DIRECTOR OF
NURSING:

Type of error. Check below:

1. ( ) Wrong medication
2. ( ) Wrong dosage
3. ( ) Wrong day/time
4. ( ) Wrong patient
5. ( ) Error in transcribing
6. ( ) Omitted medication
7. ( ) Other (Explain) _____
_____
_____

AFTER REVIEW BY HEAD NURSE
  OR SUPERVISOR SEND TO
    NURSING SERVICE
    WITHIN 24 HOURS.

SIGNATURE OF PERSON REPORTING ERROR

PERSON IN CHARGE WHEN ERROR OCCURRED

SIGNATURE OF HEAD NURSE AND/OR SUPERVISOR

Source: Adaptation of form used by Kennestone Hospital, Marietta, Georgia, 1978.

the institution's paying only medical expenses directly resulting from an incident, even though other indirect expenses were involved.
3. *Accept total responsibility.* This course may be selected when limited exposure or liability exists. Accepting all expenses involved in replacing lost dentures is an example. There may also be occasions when a significant liability potential exists; obvious negligence or fault is determined to rest with the institution. In these cases, there may be times when it is best to initially accept total responsibility. Litigation most probably would result in greater cost and exposure.
4. *Accept necessary responsibility.* This course of action is probably the most desirable in the largest number of cases. Here, the institution may start with a position of no responsibility and after discussion and negotiation accept limited responsibility or, where appropriate, even total responsibility.

The investigation techniques and the judgment necessary to arrive at the best choice of action were outlined in Chapter 2 in discussions of corrective and administrative activities. Most situations will result in a recommendation that no or only necessary responsibility be accepted, a few will call for accepting limited responsibility, and isolated cases will result in a recommendation to accept total responsibility. Of course, the severity and exposure of the incident/accident also has a bearing on the recommended resolution. Such decisions should include input from the risk manager, hospital attorney, appropriate council/committees, an administrative representative, and the insurance carrier and/or claims manager.

As a general rule, when a claim settlement is offered and accepted, an appropriate release from further liability should be obtained. The format of the release form should be tailored to the hospital's needs as well as the requirements of the specific situation. Exhibit 4-5 is an example of such a release. Though the hospital's attorney will almost always recommend obtaining such a release, the practicalities of the situation may suggest otherwise. For example, a modest (very limited responsibility) settlement is offered and accepted and seems to satisfy a potentially significant liability problem. A dogmatic request for a signature on a release form may aggravate the problem and sabotage the initial agreement. In such a case, judgment again plays a major role. The pros and cons of any action taken need to be evaluated and calculated carefully throughout the entire process.

General Problems

The second purpose of review and analysis of incident/accident reports is the determination of general trends and patterns that may be developing. The use of special forms, such as the incident report monthly summary (Exhibit

Exhibit 4-5 Release from Liability

I, _____, have received

$_____ for payment of services or losses necessitated

by an incident occurring while in or around _____

hospital.

I recognize this payment (indicate if joint payment with physician

involved) as total compensation for the incident (describe incident and date of

occurrence); and do hereby release the hospital (and physician) of further

liability.

_____   _____
Signature   Witness

_____
Type Name

_____   _____
Date   Notary Public

Source: Adaptation of form used by Kennestone Hospital, Marietta, Georgia, 1978.

4–6), can be helpful for this purpose. Categorizing and tabulating basic data will assist in identifying problem areas as well as detecting trends in the types of occurrences. Frequency of incidents should be determined, and then the severity of those incidents. The cumulative effect on the patient (or others) should be gauged, insofar as this is possible.[12] In addition, the data base should include:

- areas of the hospital where incidents are frequent (for example, emergency department)
- medical specialties and procedures that result in claims more frequently than most (for example, anesthesiology or surgery)

- situations that appear to be associated with claims (for example, improper instructions upon discharge or incomplete medical records)
- sources of information concerning the possible liability (for example, medical audit, incident report, and so forth)[13]

In addition to basic summary reports, additional analysis involving a specific type of incident/accident may be completed. Generally, this work is performed by an appropriate committee within the Council on Safety and Loss Control. An example of such an analysis dealing specifically with falls sustained by patients or the public is illustrated in Exhibit 4-7.

In this example, several interesting discoveries were made. First, the occurrences were evenly distributed over the three work shifts. Second, older persons seemed to be more prone to falls (43.1 percent were 66 years of age or older). Third, of the known causes, "falls due to medical conditions" was the most prevalent. Fourth, two or three units seemed to have more of these incidents than others.

A similar analysis was performed on incidents involving visitors' falls. An interesting outgrowth of this review: several visitors had suffered from falls in the same unit of the hospital during a single week. These occurrences were in several adjoining rooms and these persons had apparently "fainted" while visiting patients on that unit. A physical inspection of this area resulted in determining that the average temperature in these rooms was 5 to 8 degrees higher than recommended levels. This resulted from several defective thermostats that were subsequently replaced. Evidently, the patients in the rooms, who were elderly, were fairly comfortable in an elevated room temperature and had not complained.

Corrective action in response to these analyses as well as to all such situational reviews should be the end result of such efforts by the institution's risk management program.

LITIGATION PREPARATION

The ultimate stage in the resolution of any incident or accident is courtroom action in the form of conventional proceedings, arbitration, or other tort processes that may apply in different states. Traditionally, most situations are solved before reaching this stage. However, for a multitude of reasons, some problems will only be resolved in the legal forum. The final decision on the part of an individual to sue the hospital or its agents will be altered from time to time by circumstances. A display of determination on the part of the hospital to fight to the bitter end or willingness to settle out of court are two circumstances that may affect an individual's decision to sue.

Exhibit 4-6 Incident Report Monthly Summary

Area	Patient Falls	Fires	Treatment Errors	Medication Errors and Omissions	Thefts	Lost or Broken Articles	Procedural Errors	Equip. Malfunc-tion	Missing Surgical Devices	Missing Drugs	**Other
Operating Room											
Recovery Room											
Emergency Room											
Nursing Administration											
Quality Assurance											
6 North (Gen. Medical)											
6 West (Pediatrics)											
6 South (Medical/Oncology)											
5 North (Neurology)											
5 West (Orthopedics)											
5 South (Thoracic Surg.)											
4 North (Gen. Surgery)											
4 West (Gen. Medical)											
4 South (Gen. Surgery)											
PCCU (Progressive Coronary)											
CCU (Coronary Care)											

ICU (Intensive Care)
Obstetrics
Gyn (Gynecology)
Nursery
Mental Health
Rehab. Nursing
Delivery Room
I.V. Therapy
Clinic
Admissions
Outpatient Dept.
X-ray/Radiation Therapy
Laboratory
Rehab. Medicine
Nuclear Medicine
Diagnostic Imaging
Miscellaneous
TOTALS
Public Liability

Source: Adaptation of form used by Kennestone Hospital, Marietta, Georgia, 1978.

Exhibit 4-7 Analysis of Patient/Public Falls

January–December 1977

TOTAL FALLS REPORTED 561

TIMES OF OCCURRENCE	Incidents	Percentage
Day 33%		
7 a.m.–11 a.m.	105	19
11 a.m.–3 a.m.	77	14
Evening 33%		
3 p.m.–7 p.m.	91	16
7 p.m.–11 p.m.	98	17
Morning 34%		
11 p.m.–3 a.m.	95	17
3 a.m.–7 a.m.	95	17

MALE VS. FEMALE

Female—304   Male—157

AGE IN YEARS	Incidents	Percentage
0–25	65	12
26–45	104	18
46–65	150	27
66–Over	242	43

MONTH OF OCCURRENCE	
January	53
February	53
March	57
April	42
May	50
June	40
July	57
August	52
September	31
October	51
November	45
December	30

DAY OF WEEK	
Monday	78
Tuesday	88
Wednesday	85
Thursday	87
Friday	79
Saturday	78
Sunday	66

KNOWN CAUSES	Incidents	Percentage
Liquid Spills/Ice	31	5
Tripping & Slipping	69	12
Falls from bed	95	17
Falls due to medical condition	266	47
Found on floor (No known reason)	60	11
Others	40	7

DEPARTMENTS	Incidents	Percentage
4 North	44	8
4 South	30	5
4 West	86	15
5 North	77	14
5 South	24	4
5 West	46	8
6 North	63	1
6 South	5	1
6 West	26	5
ICU	7	1
CCU	3	5
PCCU	46	8
OB	6	1
GYN	10	2
Mental Health	37	7
Rehab	16	3
Others	35	6.5

TYPE OF INJURIES RECEIVED	Incidents	Percentage
Back	12	2
Hip	29	5
Leg or ankle	21	4
Arm	45	8
Knee	31	5
Laceration/Abrasion	91	16
No injury	357	60

AVERAGE EMERGENCY ROOM CHARGE WAIVED PER INCIDENT $32.50

Source: Minutes of the Patient and Public Safety Committee, Kennestone Hospital, Marietta, Georgia, February 1978.

In regard to litigation, good judgment and strategy on the part of both the hospital and its legal counsel in choosing the stance that should be taken are imperative. The quality of preparation for the legal battle is usually the key to the ultimate outcome of any case.

Since this author has no formal training nor does he claim expertise in hospital law, this section will be devoted to litigation preparation from the hospital administrator's viewpoint. Here, basic principles from an administrative perspective are suggested.

1. *Insure that factual comprehensive documentation is accomplished.* One of the primary tools that a hospital's legal counsel needs in preparation for a courtroom battle is a file full of well-documented facts. The confidential and privileged nature of the attorney–client relationship can be used in the accumulation process. As mentioned in Chapter 3, incident/accident reports with supporting information should be forwarded immediately to the hospital attorney. The timeliness of information gathering is directly related to the accuracy and caliber of facts obtained. When any incident/accident occurs, the process of preparing for a potential day in court should start. The risk management program can greatly assist in creating this conscious attitude toward possible repercussions on the part of all parties who may be involved in or are knowledgeable of a risk situation.

2. *Remember that subsequent review and analysis can also provide insight from a legal standpoint.* The activities of committees in regard to evaluation of both individual and general risk problems can be most helpful to legal counsel. The deviation from recognized standards of any incident is generally discovered during the review and analysis stage. This is significant, since one of the main criteria used in establishing the liability of a hospital is often the prevailing standard in the professional community. The practical expertise of those involved in committee work can be very helpful in establishing and evaluating the hospital's position on and approach to a given problem situation.

3. *Thorough orientation and education of the attorney relative to the technical and operational aspects of the problem situation are necessary.* It should be remembered that most attorneys are members of the laity relative to hospital activities. In this regard, it is important that the hospital's legal counsel be given a quick course in the technical aspects of the incident/accident. Capable attorneys are very adept at this and can often amaze one with their fast learning abilities. This imparted knowledge is not only important from the standpoint of preparation but also necessary in the course of the proceedings within the courtroom. The many turns and directions that a case may take can only be handled by an informed, well-versed attorney.

4. *Active participation by the hospital's governing body and administration in judgmental and strategic decisions is desirable.* At times, there may be a tendency to have the hospital attorney shoulder the entire burden when decisions need to be made in the course of litigation activities. This can be very unfair to the counsel; more important, an excellent intellectual resource may go untapped. The viewpoint of the hospital's governing and operational representatives needs to be incorporated in the decision-making process. For example, the selection of witnesses who will take the stand for the institution needs to be made carefully. The knowledge of administrators, who work daily with hospital personnel, concerning potential witnesses' abilities to handle pressure situations, their temperament, and their other capabilities can be very helpful in the final selection of witnesses.

5. *Flexibility should be maintained throughout the entire litigation process.* In the course of battle, particularly a legal one, emotions usually rise and positions often harden. Despite these tendencies, an attitude of equitable compromise should always be maintained. The high principles and integrity of the institution should always be protected; of course, these may from time to time need to be flavored a bit by reality and practicality. Decisions should always be influenced by what will be best for the hospital. Neither the pride of the governing body or administrative staff nor the ego of the hospital's legal counsel should ever serve as a deterrent to this aim.

To repeat, these priniciples relating to the litigation process primarily reflect an administrative viewpoint. It goes without saying that the most important factors assuring the hospital's legal well-being are probably the competence and savvy of the hospital legal counsel. The best legal expertise available is essential to hospitals in these trying days. The hospital's track record in the courtroom will often have a direct bearing on future exploitation of risk situations by other plaintiffs and their attorneys.

CONCLUSION

Inherent in any business or service that deals with human lives is the risk of experiencing potential liability problems. This fact must be recognized and faced as a part of organizational life, particularly in a hospital. In such a setting, an organizational sin possibly greater than the *commission* of a potentially liable incident is the *omission* of proper handling of the incident after it occurs.

The effectiveness an organization displays in handling problems does not occur by chance. To create an environment conducive to good problem solving, conscious, positive effort is necessary. An atmosphere where defined authority and responsibility exist along with a sense of accountability is very important. In addition to its normal problem-solving function, risk management should contribute significantly to the creation of this atmosphere within a hospital.

HANDLING OF POTENTIAL PROBLEMS CHECKLIST

___ Does an effective system exist to identify problem situations?

___ Is there a process of screening and determining the seriousness of each problem?

___ Do review, analysis, and resolution take place as part of the system?

___ Do follow-up procedures correct or eliminate incident / accident causes?

___ Is there a consciousness of possible litigation resulting from problems and necessary means of preparation for that possible eventuality?

Identification of problems

___ Are appropriate means established and understood for reporting problems by members of the hospital's staff?

___ Does adequate documentation occur when a problem is identified?

Incidents and accidents

___ Does a clear definition of problems (incidents) involving patients, visitors, and the general public exist?

___ Does a clear definition of problems (accidents) involving employees exist?

___ Are incident and accident report forms available and used properly?

___ Are comprehensive policies and procedures relative to the handling of incidents and accidents formulated and followed?

___ Do these policies and procedures incorporate definitions of responsibility and authority?

Centralization of information
___ Does the hospital have a systematic method of centrally recording and maintaining incidents and accidents?
___ Does the risk manager administer this program?
___ Do basic logging systems for incidents and accidents exist?

Screening process
___ Are incident/accident reports separated in major and minor categories?
___ Do major incidents/accidents receive priority in terms of review and follow-up?
___ Does the hospital attorney receive copies of all major incident/accident reports and support information?
___ Is a determination made as to the attitude of those effected by the incident/accident?
___ Are strategy and judgment used in choosing the hospital's representative to contact those involved?
___ Are these persons versed in ways of best handling the contact?

Review, analysis, and recommendations
___ Are adequate special purpose forms available to assist in the review and analysis of problem situations?
___ Are the choices of action in the resolution of individual problems understood and considered?
___ Are good investigative techniques and judgment used to determine the best course of action?
___ When settlements are made, are release forms generally signed?
___ Are general problems in terms of trends and patterns identified, addressed, and resolved?
___ Does an adequate system of review and analysis exist within the committee structure?

Litigation preparation
___ Does factual comprehensive documentation that can be used in litigation preparation generally exist in most risk situations?
___ Are review and analysis reports available for use by the hospital's legal counsel?

___ Is the hospital attorney thoroughly oriented in the technical and operational aspects of problem situations that must be litigated?

___ Do the governing body and administration participate in judgmental and strategic decision making?

___ Is a position of flexibility maintained throughout the litigation process?

Note: This checklist is not meant to be all-inclusive nor does it require absolute adherence. Its purpose is to stimulate thought and redirect attitudes toward the establishment of a risk management program.

NOTES

1. C. Epting, "Of Mice and Men: Health Risks and Safety Judgments," *Facts and Issues, League of Women Voters, 1977,* p. 1.

2. J. Ashby, S. Stephens, and S. Pearson, "Elements in Successful Risk Reduction Programs," *Hospital Progress,* July 1977, p. 62.

3. G. Newman, "Basic Elements of a Loss Control Program," *Hospital Progress,* November 1974, p. 49.

4. T. Dankmyer and J. Groves, "Taking Steps for Safety's Sake," *Hospitals, JAHA,* May 16, 1977, p. 61.

5. S. Holloway and A. Sax, "AHA Urges, Aids Hospitals to Adopt Effective Risk Management Plans," *Hospitals, JAHA* May 16, 1977, p. 58.

6. B. Passett, "Education Can Help Control Hospital Liability," *Cross-Reference,* May/June 1977, p. 5.

7. *Controlling Hospital Liability: A Systems Approach,* developed and written by the Maryland Hospital Education Institute (Chicago, Ill.: American Hospital Association, 1976), p. 4.

8. *Log of Occupational Injuries and Illnesses,* OSHA No. 200.

9. *Controlling Hospital Liability: A Systems Approach,* p. 15.

10. M. Grayson, "Risk Management: New Focus for Traditional Functions," *The Hospital Medical Staff,* May 1978, p. 14.

11. S. Rothman, "Hospital Goes Bare," *Risk Management,* November 16, 1976, p. 70.

12. T. Dankmyer and J. Groves, p. 62.

13. *Controlling Hospital Liability: A Systems Approach,* p. 15.

Chapter 5

Program Justification and Feasibility

The decision to institute any new hospital program in today's cost-conscious environment usually must be supported by a feasibility study and a cost-justification analysis. A risk management program should be viewed in the same manner, although certain inherent weaknesses will prevent drawing a totally accurate picture.

Risk management has many of the same intangible and subjective characteristics that are found in most other *staff* services. First, the program is not a revenue or income producer; it is, instead, a cost-saving function. At times, cost-saving activities are more difficult to justify fiscally than are revenue-producing ones. This is particularly true if the projected savings are not hard and definitive in nature. Second, cost savings and other benefits resulting from the program's efforts are normally reflected in other departments' operations. This is principally the case because staff activities are by nature supportive of and advisory to other functions within the organization. Finally, the true cost of a staff program is very difficult to measure since so much of its activity, again by nature, indirectly involves other departments within the hospital. Committee work, report preparation, statistical accumulation and analysis, and follow-up activities by representatives throughout the organization are examples of this unmeasurable involvement. A significant difference exists between the direct, measurable cost and the total cost of a program such as this.

When other staff functions, such as personnel and public relations departments, were initially conceived, they probably suffered from many of the same difficulties in regard to feasibility determination and cost justification. However, these and other staff functions have proved their worth, in spite of their impalpable nature. Risk management may have a greater potential than many of these existing staff programs for two main reasons: (1) the cost resulting from institutional liability (including potential loss) is exceedingly high in most hospitals, and, therefore, a significant possibility exists for cost savings; (2) so many of the activities in the risk management function already exist and only need redirection and coordination, which, hopefully, can be accomplished with limited financial outlay.

FACTORS INVOLVED IN DETERMINATION

Because each hospital is unique, the decision to venture into any new activity will vary from one institution to another. Regardless of institutional idiosyncrasies, certain common factors need to be considered in determining the direction a hospital will take relative to a risk management program. These factors will significantly influence not only the decision to enact a program but also the form that it ultimately takes. The list includes:

- type of insurance program currently in force
- size and scope of the hospital
- risk history and experience
- community attitudes
- patient, public, and employee demographics

Type of Insurance Program

As previously mentioned, some of the risk management functions may be delegated to an insurance carrier as part of the hospital's insurance program. Safety, education, and claim surveillance and management are examples of such activities. In determining the feasibility of a formal internal risk management program, existing functions handled externally need to be taken into consideration. Unnecessary duplication and/or conflicting functions need to be avoided because they will adversely affect attempts to justify the cost of a program. If the hospital desires to take over or appropriately supplement some of the risk management activities currently offered under its insurance program, a possible savings in premiums can be realized through discussion and negotiations with the insuring agent. Though not widespread or prevalent as yet, this approach would be comparable to the preferential rating system used in automobile insurance under *good driver* and *driver education* plans.

If the hospital is self-insured, the need automatically exists for a comprehensive risk management program. In addition, to the humane and financial reasons for having such a program, a hospital under a self-insurance plan must have a risk management program to meet requirements for participation in Medicare. According to Medicare regulations, each hospital must have an adequate risk management program to examine the cause of losses and to take action to reduce the frequency and severity of them. A hospital must have an ongoing safety program, professional and employee training programs, etc., to minimize the frequency and severity of malpractice and comprehensive general patient liability incidents.[1]

Size and Scope of the Hospital

The size as well as the scope of patient services offered within the hospital will also contribute significantly to the need for formalizing risk management activities. Naturally, the exposure to risk and potential liability increases as a hospital's patient load grows. As number of admissions, patient days, and outpatient/emergency room visits increase, many more opportunities for risk problems come into being.

The scope of the services offered in the institution also will increase risk potential. A modern hospital offers a broad array of services that potentially carry greater risk (e.g., emergency service, operating room, and intensive care). Additionally, many highly specialized services (e.g., cardiovascular, thoracic, plastic and neurosurgery, gynecology, and high-risk nurseries) tend to present risk problems.

Risk History and Experience

Any new program more easily justifies itself in hospitals where an obvious problem exists that may be eliminated or at least alleviated by the new program. A comprehensive risk management program may initially be more appealing to hospitals with poor track records relative to liability cost than to hospitals that feel relatively secure in regard to this problem. Costs that already exist are looked upon as prime targets for any program aimed at cost reduction, whereas the reduction of *potential* costs is often less dramatic as a program objective. Even though a hospital's history in regard to malpractice and other liability cost is favorable, the good record should not serve as a reason for discounting the feasibility of a risk management program. An institution with a good record will only retain such status by being progressive in its management and operational activities. Risk management, if appropriately conceived and developed, has the potential of being such a progressive activity in all hospital settings.

Community Attitudes

Malpractice exposure has reached epidemic levels in certain parts of the country while other regions have experienced far fewer cases. This fact will influence some in regard to a risk management program in their hospitals. There is a natural tendency to act when problems are imminent and to defer action when they are not. But remember that epidemics tend to spread rapidly. As the old saying goes, *an ounce of prevention is worth a pound of cure.* There are many examples of contagious trends, such as the acceleration of health care costs, increased unionization, crime rate growth, and unemployment and inflation levels. Trends that originate in one part of the country tend to move eventually into other areas. However, in the short run, regional and community attitudes directly influence liability cost and therefore influence feasibility of programs geared to reducing such cost.

Demographics

In determining the market for a product or the feasibility of a service, demographic criteria play a significant part. *Demographic segmentation* is a term used to describe the process of evaluating those characteristics. These demographic criteria usually include:

- sex
- age
- marital status
- income
- ethnic factors
- education
- geographic location
- occupation[2]

It may seem obvious how criteria such as these influence the marketability of such new product items as food, clothing and furniture, but one may ask, "What does this have to do with a risk management program?" Well, a little perceptive thinking will lead one to see the relevance of such a program within the hospital setting. A few examples may help to make this clearer:

1. Sex: Studies have indicated that surgical procedures involving the female genital system result in the largest percentage of paid claims as compared to other surgery.[3] Therefore, the sex composition of the hospital patient population directly affects potential claims.
2. *Age:* The analysis of patient falls cited in Chapter 4 indicated that a significantly greater number of such incidents involved older people (aged 60 or over). Therefore, age may also have a direct relationship to frequency of certain incidents.
3. *Income:* Incidents resulting in injury or disability to those at high income levels provide greater risk exposure. A technique often used in the courtroom when seeking large judgments against a hospital is to define personal worth based on an individual's potential lifetime income. Educational and occupational levels of patients may tend to have a similar effect.

4. *Geographic location:* This has already been cited earlier under community attitudes.

Employee demography plays a similar role relative to workmen's compensation risks. The hospital's patient/public/employee composition does influence even a negative product market, such as risk within a hospital setting, and should be considered in justification of the risk management program.

BUDGET FORMULATION

This author once worked for a man who began by asking one basic question when evaluating any activity. This question was, "What is the bottom line?" He was an outstanding administrator. Few, if any, inappropriate and unjustified programs ever came into existence in his organization. A means of determining the bottom line, to the degree possible, of a risk management program, begins with the formulation of the budget. Realizing that there are many types of budgets, including operating, capital, cash, and long- and short-term (and probably more), the term *budget* here is used in a general operational sense. In this context, it is defined as the plan that management expects to carry out expressed in financial terms—a system by which management can continuously evaluate results against goals and expectations.[4]

Certain prerequisites necessary to the establishment of a budgetary system exist and because of this necessity should be given consideration in the budgetary process for programs such as risk management. These prerequisites are:

1. A set of well-defined policies and objectives
2. A sound organizational structure, including involvement by all levels of management
3. A responsible accounting system
4. A functionally classified system of accounts
5. The accumulation of adequate statistical data, incorporating knowledge of significant trends
6. An established budgetary fiscal year
7. A formal reporting system[5]

The budget of any function is affected directly by the size and scope of the program. Therefore, it possibly would be helpful to develop several hypothetical operational budgets for risk management programs ranging from small to large in size and scope. These are illustrated in Exhibit 5–1.

Exhibit 5-1 Risk Management Program Annual Budget

	Small	Medium	Large
Salaries and benefits:			
Risk manager	$3,000*	$15,000**	$25,000***
Secretarial and clerical	4,000	8,000	17,000
Outside services:			
Consultant fees	2,000	4,000	4,000
Legal fees (related directly to program	5,000	5,000	5,000
Supplies and expense:	2,000	3,000	4,000
Indirect expense	3,000	4,000	5,000
Total	$19,000	$39,000	$60,000

*Existing department head given additional responsibilities for the program.
**Part-time and/or untrained risk manager with development potential.
***Full-time experienced risk manager.

Note: These budgets are based on prevailing cost in the Southeast; should be adjusted for regional differences.

Of course, budgets should be kept in perspective, for they must also relate directly to the purposes and objectives of a program. Additionally, a philosophy of management by objectives as part of the budgeting process can significantly contribute to the attainment of goals intended for any program.[6] (See the section, Managing Risk by Objectives, Chapter 6.) These hypothetical examples of budgets naturally lack specific defined purposes and objectives for the risk management programs. From a practical standpoint, they can only serve as a basic guide to and frame of reference for budget development for individual hospitals contemplating a risk management function.

Relating to Total Liability Costs

To gain a better perspective of the cost of risk management, this cost as it relates to other liability expenses influenced by an effective risk management program needs to be thoroughly considered. This exercise is commonly used in reviewing and evaluating other management functions. For example, general administrative and financial management costs are often viewed as a percentage of total operating cost, personnel administration cost is related to total payroll and other personnel-related expense, and department management cost is considered as a percentage of total departmental operating cost. In other words, the use of a relative factor or denominator may give a more positive view of the potential cost and ultimate worth of an organizational activity. If management costs of a program are relatively low and potential savings attributed to the program are relatively high, feasibility is enhanced.

In the case of risk management, the cost of the program should be related to those total direct expenses associated with losses due to institutional liability that could possibly feel the impact of a risk management program. Some of these costs include:

- general and professional liability insurance premiums or the cost associated with a self-insurance plan
- workman's compensation premiums
- other casualty insurance premiums
- hospitalization insurance premiums (related to job injury or illness)
- deductibles on insurance programs
- additional legal and consultant fees related to liability cases
- related leave expense
- expenses such as minor claim settlements, related courtesy discounts, and the like
- excessive rates or escalating cost of the above
- other related cost that may be identified by the hospital

When these costs are totaled, a significant dollar amount usually results. If the estimated cost of the proposed risk management program is evaluated in terms of a percentage of these overall risk-related expenses, a new perspective on the establishment of the program is gained. For example, if the total of these costs amounts to $600,000 and the projected annual budget for the risk management program is $30,000, then a 5 percent direct investment is being made and directed toward reducing the overall real cost of liability. Of course, this is a dramatic example that demonstrates significant potential relative to program feasibility. It will not always be that obvious. Also, it should be noted that although indirect costs and benefits were not included in the foregoing list, empirical knowledge would lead one to expect even further justification of the risk management program when these factors are considered.

RISK MANAGEMENT AS A SERVICE

As mentioned initially, the feasibility and justification of the risk management program should not be viewed from a financial angle alone. Another and equally important consideration is the *service* provided by such an activity.

In some cases, the decision to formalize a risk management program is an obvious one and is easily justified. However, in most situations, this determination may be much more difficult to make when considering only the financial aspects. It is in these instances that the hospital must consider its social responsibility when making the decision of whether to proceed or not. Concern about immediate profit (or cost savings) makes it rather difficult to invest in areas where profits cannot be accurately measured and where the returns are long run in nature.[7]

Some will argue that a social responsibility exists in all organizations, particularly in institutions providing human services, such as hospitals. Generally, "social responsibility" is used to refer to areas ranging from the quality and safety of an organization's product to cures for current social problems.[8] This philosophy, if subscribed to, will reinforce certain institutional policies which, in themselves, are not always cost justified. Management decisions and actions taken for reasons at least partially beyond the organization's direct economic or technical interest are defined as social responsibility.[9]

John P. Schmitt, in an article entitled "Risk Management Justification: Cost-Benefit Considerations,"[10] suggested that most risk management programs could not be totally justified on a cost basis. In addition, he emphasized the institution's social responsibility. Nonfinancial benefits potentially available as a result of an effective program include:

- an improved reputation for patient care
- improved compliance with accreditation and safety requirements (e.g., incident reporting system, safety orientation for new employees, establishment of a reference library dealing with all facets of hospital safety)[11]
- enhanced intraorganizational communication among committees (e.g., safety committee, infection control committee, education committee)

Hospital management teams, as guardians of the community's health care resources, must structure their risk management program in accordance with their organization's primary mission, quality patient care. Economic results cannot be neglected, but they must be viewed as secondary outcomes that can be optimized only within the parameters of acceptable standards of treatment.[12]

CONCLUSION

Another administrator, with whom this author is familiar, uses a basic rule when determining an organizational direction on different issues that seem to be clouded by many unknowns. He asks this question: "What will this do for the patient?" If this same question is asked about a risk management program, some encouraging answers come to light: It will provide a safer environment, it will correct problem situations to prevent recurrences, it will reinforce positive attitudes among hospital staffs, and it will create a better sense of confidence and security among the hospital's customers and consumers. These are a few of the possible answers that reflect very favorably on the program. Possibly the only negative answer that would be suggested is: it *may* cost the patient more.

From a service standpoint, a risk management program in a hospital setting is easily justified. From a financial standpoint, such a program in some form (even if limited at first) will also more than likely pass the feasibility test. The decision is, however, an individual institutional one.

JUSTIFICATION AND FEASIBILITY CHECKLIST

___ Is it understood that risk management, like other staff services, may lack tangible criteria normally used to determine feasibility and cost justification?

___ Is it understood that a risk management program is a cost saver and not a revenue producer?

___ Is the impact of the hospital's insurance program on risk management understood?

___ Is the impact of the size and scope of the hospital on the program understood?

___ Is the effect of the hospital's history and experience relative to liability cost understood?

___ Is the impact of community attitudes on the risk management program understood?

___ Are the implications of demographics on the risk management program understood?

Budget formulation

___ Is the formal budget exercise performed as part of the cost justification process?

___ Are the prerequisites necessary for a budget process considered?

___ Is a philosophy of management by objectives integrated into the budget process?

Relative to total liability costs

___ Is the risk management program cost viewed in relation to total liability costs?

___ Has total institutional liability cost been defined?

Risk management as a service

___ Does your institution subscribe to the philosophy of social responsibility?

___ Do you consider a risk management program consistent with this philosophy?

NOTES

1. *Medicare Provider Reimbursement Manual* (Washington, D.C.: USDHEW Social Security Administration, April 1977) p. 2162.3.

2. David J. Schwartz, *Marketing Today: A Basic Approach* (New York: Harcourt Brace Jovanovich, Inc., 1977), p. 82.

3. *NAIC Malpractice Claims,* Vol. 1, April 1976, p. 27.

4. G. Black, "Hospital Budgeting," unpublished manuscript, 1977, p. 6.

5. R. Baker, "Prerequisites of a Budget System," *Planning the Hospital Financial Operations: Reading in Hospital Budgeting,* Compiled by HFMA, 1972, p. 39.

6. G. Black, p. 11.

7. Leslie W. Rue and Lloyd L. Byars, *Management Theory and Application* (Homewood, Ill.: Richard D. Irwin, Inc., 1977), p. 469.

8. Ibid, pp. 463–464.

9. K. David, "Can Business Afford to Ignore Social Responsibilities?" *California Management Review,* Spring 1960, p. 70.

10. J. Schmitt, "Risk Management Justification: Cost-Benefit Considerations," *Risk Management,* July 1977, p. 42.

11. *Accreditation Manual for Hospitals* (Chicago: Joint Commission on Accreditation of Hospitals, 1976).

12. Schmitt, p. 42.

Chapter 6

A Philosophical Look at a Risk Management Program

Approaching a subject philosophically is always intriguing, for it allows an author to venture from totally factual and technical observations to personal concepts and beliefs concerning the area of interest. To this point, this book has been primarily geared to promoting the idea of risk management in a hospital setting. Such a program offers many advantages and has the potential of becoming a very positive management tool. However, for any program to be successful, some basic ingredients must be present in the organization. Some of these have been mentioned previously but warrant repetition and emphasis.

RECOGNITION OF DISEASE

Prescribing a risk management program for hospitals is analogous to prescribing medicine for patients. When patients contract infection, drugs are usually ordered as therapy; even when they are just exposed to disease, the medicine is often used for prophylactic reasons. Similarly, hospitals with obvious risk problems need immediate treatment, and even those that are exposed but not suffering may need a risk management program for prophylactic purposes.

Possibly the most important factor in the elimination or at least alleviation of organizational disease is a recognition by the organization that an ailment exists. As in physical illness, the first indications of organizational disease are usually symptoms. Symptoms of risk/liability problems may or may not be obvious ones. Such indications as dramatically rising insurance premiums and liability claims are immediately apparent, whereas latent safety hazards, substandard professional practices, and negative attitudes are sometimes less distinguishable yet very real symptoms of chronic risk disease. A routine examination on a regular basis is usually the recommended approach to good physical health. The same approach will also serve as an excellent deterrent for acute organizational disease in the area of risk problems and liability losses. (The prerequisites for a risk management program described in Chapter 2 will serve as a form for conducting a risk examination in the hospital setting.)

COMMITMENT TO PRODUCE RESULTS

History has demonstrated that it is popular to foster new programs and activities but very unpopular to discontinue them once established. This is a bureaucratic tendency from which most hospitals suffer. For this reason, it is important that a new function be not only properly conceived but also committed from the beginning to produce results. Time and time again, new activities that have been added to the hospital directory of services under the guise of cost reduction and efficiency promotion prove to be something to the contrary. A formal risk management program should not be incorporated in a hospital just because others are doing it. It should only come into existence for a specific purpose and objective: eliminating and reducing organizational risk and associated cost through a management program.

The need to look at cost/benefit considerations of hospital risk management programs is a first step in program justification. Unless some effort is made to bridge the gap of understanding between economic investment and tangible and intangible returns, however, hospital risk managers may find themselves hard put to explain the purpose of their programs to top management, patients, and their facilities' health care communities.[1]

MANAGING RISK BY OBJECTIVES

A technique that comes as close as any to measuring the effectiveness of an organizational activity is management by objectives (MBO). The MBO process varies among institutions that have used it successfully, but the purpose is the same. Basically, it requires those organizationally involved to participate in defining the following components:

1. Statement of function or purpose
2. Short- and long-term accomplishments realized during past reporting periods
3. Short- and long-term measurable objectives for future reporting periods
4. Resources (personnel quotas, operating and capital budgets) necessary to fulfill the organization's purpose and meet established objectives

If accomplishments and objectives are to have meaning in truly evaluating an activity, they must be stated in measurable terms. Too often MBO documents include only statements of goals, such as "promote patient safety," "increase efficiency and productivity," and "improve employee morale." Even though these certainly are and should be functional objectives, they need to be stated in reasonable, definite terms that can be measured. For example, in regard to patient safety, here are a few specific objectives.

1. Develop and conduct a course on fire safety to be attended by all employees.
2. Review and update all policies and procedures related to safety during the next year.
3. Conduct a slogan-of-the-month contest on safety.
4. Organize and conduct safety orientation program for all new employees. . . .

Charles G. Lenhard, in an article entitled "Building a Result Oriented Control Program," stated:

> Not only should the program be obvious throughout the hospital, but it also must be able to be measured. It is important to evaluate the effectiveness of the control program regularly. . . . formal, written, well articulated risk control program, complete with stated goals and specified criteria for evaluation, demonstrates a hospital's unwillingness to leave incidents and claims' outcomes to chance.[2]

If the benefits arising from the risk management program are to be quantified, the focus must be on the hospital performance/patient (and others, including employees and visitors) state of health relationship. Therefore, the optimal benefit to the patient and all others offered by the risk management program can be deemed the insurance that proper treatment will be given without variation from prescribed routine.[3]

ORGANIZATIONAL ACCEPTANCE

In tradition-saturated organizations, such as hospitals, new and different programs can be formally accepted by edict, yet informally rejected by apathy. The methods used to establish such programs often have a profound effect on true organizational acceptance.

This author had an interesting experience recently in a major hospital building program. For the first time in this particular institution, department heads were asked to become intimately involved in the concept and design planning stages relative to their new departments. This process of involvement required much more time, education, discussion, and negotiation than had been necessary in previous building programs. The result was a more functional facility and a true commitment on the part of operational managers to make the new facility work to its maximum potential. A creative sense of pride existed and has had a positive effect on organizational effectiveness and efficiency.

This experience leads one to believe that the establishment of all new activities should include maximum organizational involvement at the outset. In the case of risk management, initial efforts made to obtain input by appropriate members of the team will pay impressive dividends in the long run in terms of the program's productivity. It has been mentioned several times that the commitment of top administration is necessary, but overall organizational acceptance and support is also an indispensable requirement.

AGAIN, STAFF MANAGEMENT

This author has mentioned and emphasized that risk management is a staff *service* and a management *function*. However, because staff management is unique in nature and requires different talents and abilities, additional explanation seems appropriate.

Probably the best example of a staff manager is an executive secretary to a chief executive officer of a large organization. A person filling the position has a tremendous amount of responsibility, not only to handle routine clerical and secretarial activities but also the overall work flow within the office. This, in turn, affects almost every area of the organization. A request received, action taken, response given, and problems solved are often contingent upon good staff work performed by the executive secretary. Interestingly, this person does not usually have the formal authority commensurate with responsibility, yet the job must be done.

Both the risk manager and the risk management function fit into the same *staff management* category. A significant responsibility exists, yet often formal authority to enact and expedite needed activities may be lacking. To counter this inherent characteristic of a program such as risk management, its manager must develop an operational repertoire that includes, in addition to normal administrative skills, such tools as finesse, diplomacy, reconciliation, a sense of humor, and the bluff. The important thing is that risk management in the hospital become effective, and the use of unusual management skills may be necessary to accomplish the program's purposes and objectives.

CONCLUSION

The mere existence of a program such as risk management in a hospital has a certain psychological effect upon the organization similar to the effect of a self-insurance program. The emphasis given to such activities as safety, security, patient and public relations, and other functions closely identified with loss prevention no doubt influences the attitudes and actions of both the providers and the recipients of care in the hospital.

A good doctor–patient relationship has been proved to be one of the best deterrents to liability claims against physicians.[4] Likewise, a hospital's own bedside manner reflected in its relations with patients is probably its greatest weapon in claims prevention. The promotion of good will, friendliness, concern, and helpfulness should go hand in hand with competence, quality, and effectiveness as primary aims of an institution. A risk management program will not take the place of these, but it will enhance and supplement such institutional characteristics. Risk management is not *the* answer to liability problems, but it can be *part* of the solution.

RISK MANAGEMENT PHILOSOPHY CHECKLIST

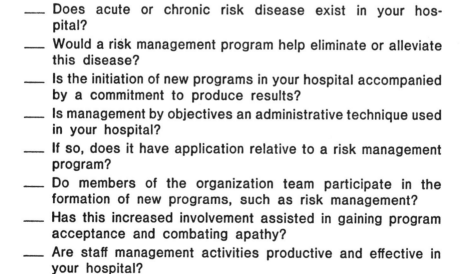

___ Does acute or chronic risk disease exist in your hospital?

___ Would a risk management program help eliminate or alleviate this disease?

___ Is the initiation of new programs in your hospital accompanied by a commitment to produce results?

___ Is management by objectives an administrative technique used in your hospital?

___ If so, does it have application relative to a risk management program?

___ Do members of the organization team participate in the formation of new programs, such as risk management?

___ Has this increased involvement assisted in gaining program acceptance and combating apathy?

___ Are staff management activities productive and effective in your hospital?

___ Does your hospital have a good bedside manner?

NOTES

1. J. Schmitt, "Risk Management Justification: Cost/Benefit Considerations," *Risk Management,* July 1977, p. 40.

2. C. Lenhard, "Building a Result Oriented Control Program," *Risk Management,* July 1977, p. 18.

3. Schmitt, p. 40.

4. "Patient/Physician Communication Helps Avoid Malpractice Suits," *The Blue Shield News,* February 1978, p. 6.

Chapter 7

Self-Insurance

As recorded in a published article by Bernard M. Brown, there are four major options for hospitals relative to professional liability loss exposures.[1] These are:

1. *Commercial insurance* or purchased insurance program from a commercial insurance carrier
2. *Joint Underwriting Association* (JUA) to force commercial insurers to provide liability insurance to hospitals and others unable to obtain insurance (The JUA acts as an underwriting agent for the commercial underwriters or, alternatively, may reinsure existing policies of underwriters who do not wish to accept business.)
3. *Captive insurance* or different organizations, usually in the same industry, forming a captive insurance company through the pooling of risk premiums and cost
4. *Self-insurance* or retaining risk within the organization and providing a funding mechanism to cover cost

Self-insurance is probably the most recent option to become popular in hospitals. It has long been used by many manufacturing or other service organizations, particularly in the area of workmen's compensation and property risks.[2]

The term *self-insurance* is one of the most misused in insurance today. In reality, self-insurance means the recognition of an exposure to loss, a critical evaluation of risk as to the possible and probable frequency and severity of an occurrence as determined by the actuarial sciences, and financial decisions as to how best to minimize the cost of risk. A distinguishing aspect of a self-insurance program is the funding mechanism. Alternative solutions include the funding of possible losses from current income, sinking funds, lines of credit with banks, restricted trust, and other such means.[3]

A decision to self-insure is a difficult one for most hospitals. As long as the institution has the more conventional type of insurance program in existence, it is able to transfer all or part of the liability risks with which it may be faced. There is a certain degree of comfort in being insured by another party. Additionally, conscientious hospital trustees are generally cautious in regard to decisions that they feel may in any way adversely reflect on the fulfillment of their fiduciary responsibilities. In good faith, they desire to be above criticism and to avoid unnecessary personal as well as institutional exposure to it. However, containment of insurance costs has become so important to hospital trustees and executives that the former attitude of cover-it-and-forget-it has been replaced by a new philosophy and a more mature treatment called risk management.[4]

It should be remembered that a risk management program is not contingent upon being self-insured. Such a program should be considered, irrespective of the type of insurance carried by the hospital. However, the decision to self-insure usually precipitates immediate initiation of a risk management program.

According to the American Hospital Association, although risk management should be pursued by all hospitals, it is especially important for hospitals that use self-insuring mechanisms to incorporate risk management activities into their self-insurance programs.[5] This is desirable for two reasons. First, risk prevention activities, both by reducing the possibility that patients will be harmed during their hospitalization and by providing for increased visitor, employee, and physical plant safety can, in the long run, produce cost savings for hospitals.[6,7] Second, the Medicare Bureau requires that self-insuring hospitals have risk management programs if they wish to have their fund contributions treated as allowable costs.[8]

MULTIPLE APPROACHES

There are many approaches to self-insurance for general and professional liability. Some hospitals choose to self-insure on first dollar coverage (deductible) up to a specific limit, at which time a commercial umbrella policy comes into effect. Others decide to carry a small commercial plan while providing a self-insurance umbrella. And, of course, there are those that totally self-insure. No doubt, there are other approaches not mentioned here.

It should be recognized that general and professional liability coverage cannot be easily separated. In many problem situations, a debate can occur as to the classification of liability. For example, when a particular incident occurs, a question may arise concerning cause: Was the incident caused by an equipment malfunction (general) or by poor judgment on the part of a hospital employee (professional)? Therefore, these two aspects of the liability insurance program should remain together, regardless of the insurance source selected.

When converting from a commercial to a self-insurance plan, care must be taken in identifying and understanding the liability exposure that the new program will cover. Commercial insurance policies generally cover claims on either an occurrence or claims-made basis. The extent of future liability for the self-insurance plan will be significantly influenced by the provisions of the commercial policy being discontinued. On a cancelled *occurrence* policy, future claims for prior exposure will not be the responsibility of the self-insurance plan. Cancellation of a *claims-made* policy, on the other hand, will result in immediate exposure for the new program from past occurrences of liability.

REASONS TO SELF-INSURE

The decision to enter into a self-insurance program in most cases has resulted from one or both of two reasons: first, purchased insurance is too costly; second, malpractice insurance (at any price) may not be available.[9] Some authorities do not recommend a self-insurance program for small hospitals. Bernard M. Brown indicated that generally speaking, a hospital probably should not consider a self-insurance program unless its premiums for alternative commercial insurance approximate at least $400,000 annually. Why? Simply because a hospital that pays a premium of at least $400,000 is less likely to have the premium drained away by one incident than a hospital that pays a smaller premium.[10] Another factor influencing this decision may be the current experiences with liability claims and awards of other hospitals in the geographic region. For example, the southeast has historically fared much better than the west or northeast in regard to high liability judgments, although the trend can change rapidly. The extent of potential exposure as influenced by the local risk climate may certainly influence a decision to self-insure.

NECESSARY DOCUMENTS

Generally, when a self-insurance program is established, two formal documents must be developed to meet Medicare requirements. These are (1) the *self-insurance plan,* which outlines the purpose and the specifics of how this particular program functions, and (2) the restricted *trustee agreement,* which establishes the funding mechanism for the program. (Examples of these documents are illustrated in Appendixes C and D.) While these examples deal only with a self-insurance program for general and professional liability, an expansion of this plan or separate plans may be initiated to cover other aspects of the total hospital insurance program. Also, laws in different states will influence the specifics included in such documents.

The funding level for the self-insurance plan needs to be actuarially determined and documented to receive maximum reimbursement under existing federal programs. Therefore, as required in the trust agreement, an actuarial analysis must be performed annually. The level of funding for professional liability will normally be based on such factors as basic limits of the plan, occupied beds, outpatient/emergency visits and additional related interests. In regard to general liability, such factors as size and type of facilities, parking areas, and plan limits are given prime consideration in the funding determination process. The actuarial projections will also take into consideration the experience of the hospital, the experience of all hospitals in the area, the amount and timing of loss payments, and the amount of expected investment income that will be earned in the self-insurance trust fund.[11]

One factor that has discouraged some institutions from entering into self-insurance programs is the stipulation in many outstanding hospital bond issues that adequate liability insurance will be carried with a licensed carrier.

The purpose of this requirement, usually enacted years prior to the malpractice crisis, is to protect the institution's assets to insure its ability to pay off the bond indebtedness. At the same time, most of these bond agreements and resolutions also contain a stipulation that the institution's governing body and administration operate the hospital in a fiscally prudent manner. Again, this provision seeks to insure the hospital's ability to financially retire the bonds.

Of course, the decision to make changes and the manner of implementing any changes that may affect such existing obligations and commitments as bond issues have legal implications. In addition, requirements of the institution may exist that are contradictory. For example, a hospital must satisfy the requirement to carry liability insurance. A basic general and professional plan with limits up to $1 million is considered adequate. However, the low bid on such a plan by a licensed insurance carrier is $500,000. The governing body would probably consider a decision to purchase such a plan fiscally improper. This results in a legal dilemma for the organization. It can either meet the provision to have adequate commercial insurance or fulfill the requirement to operate the hospital in a fiscally responsible manner. It cannot do both.

The hospital's legal counsel needs to take all such factors into consideration when giving opinions about a self-insurance program that, on the surface, may be contrary to verbiage in such documents as bond agreements and resolutions.

The emphasis in this chapter has been given primarily to self-insurance as it relates to the professional and general liability of the organization. However, self-insurance in other aspects of the total insurance program of the hospital is also increasing in popularity. Workmen's compensation, unemployment, hospitalization, medical, and property insurance plans have been successfully implemented in some hospitals on a self-insurance basis.

The direction that a hospital takes—transferring risk through an outside insurance program or retaining risk through a self-insurance plan—should be decided after a look at the pros and cons of each. A risk management program can serve to enhance and supplement the plan selected, regardless of which is chosen.

PSYCHOLOGY OF SELF-INSURANCE

Although a formal self-insurance program is generally founded on an actuarial funding base similar to commercial insurance, a different attitude often exists toward it within an organization. Internally, self-insurance is often viewed as lack of insurance against operational hazards. Such psychological feelings can be both advantageous and detrimental to the organization. The conscientiousness of the hospital staff may increase because of the feeling of vulnerability; at the same time, a lack of confidence in the organization may also be felt. To capitalize on the advantages and, hopefully, eliminate the detrimental feelings, the self-insurance program must be explained properly to the organization. The fact that such a plan does exist in a formal sense gives credence to its purpose and objectives. As time passes, the effectiveness of the program will make itself known. Of course, a major advantage of such a program is the lowering of cost, which properly results in benefits not only to patients but also to employees. Again, reduction in the cost of negative programs can enhance the organization's ability to provide positive ones.

From a practical standpoint, a self-insurance program has a similar psychological impact on patients or others involved in incidents/accidents. Self-insurance many times has the same connotation as *no* insurance to these individuals. The immediate tendency to make claims or sue an impersonal insurance company is obvious. However, some reluctance may exist to take similar action directed toward the community's hospital. The initial inquiry made by most victims of hospital incidents (or their agents) is the question, "Who is your insurance carrier?"

The explanation given to those making claims or threatening suit can be handled in a diplomatic manner when an honest statement can be made that the hospital cannot afford an expensive insurance policy and only has a fund to cover any problem situations. The public is very knowledgeable about the high cost of malpractice insurance because of recent publicity and should have some sympathy toward a hospital's inability to afford it.

These psychological aspects certainly should not be determining factors in choosing the route of self-insurance, but they do influence attitudes toward the hospital, both externally and internally.

CONCLUSION

Self-insurance has a good ring to some, because an implication seems to exist that some savings to the institution will result. In some cases, this no doubt will occur, but administrators should beware of false impressions. The implementation of a self-insurance plan no more guarantees savings than investment in the stock market assures a profit. To those institutions that thoroughly review such programs, adequately analyze them, and then intelligently decide to self-insure, the programs will be valuable assets; but indiscriminate action by hospitals in this direction can be disastrous if misconceived or inappropriately initiated. Hospitals' decisions in regard to their insurance programs should be totally objective ones. As with any institutional investment, hard facts, sound advice, and clear judgment and thinking are imperative.

SELF-INSURANCE CHECKLIST

___ Is conventional commercial insurance available to your hospital at reasonable cost?

___ Are you familiar with other options open to your hospital relative to liability loss exposures?

___ Are you considering a self-insurance program?

___ Do you understand the multiple approaches to a self-insurance program?

___ Do you consider your hospital large enough to enter into a self-insurance program?

___ Do you understand basic documents that must be developed for such a program?

___ Do you have legal restrictions, such as bond agreements or resolutions, that prohibit your hospital's implementing a self-insurance plan?

___ How do your employees feel about being covered under a self-insurance plan?

___ Can self-insurance be used to your hospital's advantage in countering claims?

___ Is there a basic understanding of the meaning of a self-insurance program as it might be applied in your hospital?

NOTES

1. B. M. Brown, "Malpractice Risk," *Risk Management,* July 1977, p. 25–32.

2. Ibid., p. 29.

3. J. Wood (ed.) "Risk Management," *Topics in Health Care Financing,* Vol. 1, No. 4 (Summer 1975): p. 15.

4. Ibid., p. 3.

5. A. Korsak, "Risk Management Activities Boost Effectiveness of Self Insurance Program," *Hospitals, JAHA,* February 16, 1978, p. 28.

6. J. Ashley, S. Stephens, and S. Pearson, "Elements in Successful Risk Management Programs," *Hospital Progress,* July 1977, p. 58.

7. F. Daniel, "From Charitable Immunity to Public Accountability: A Review of Selected Solutions to the Malpractice Problems." *Topics in Health Care Financing,* Vol. 3, No. 4 (Summer 1977): p. 32.

8. B. Welch, "Self-Insurance: An Area Approach to Solving the Malpractice Problem," *Hospitals, JAHA,* September 16, 1977, p. 82.

9. S. Takahashi, "Self Insurance: Can It Be a Viable Alternative in the Crisis," *FAH Review,* February 1977, p. 43.

10. B. M. Brown, "Malpractice Risk Financing: New Options Complicate a Once Easy Decision," *Trustee,* December 1977, p. 40.

11. Ibid., p. 39.

Chapter 8

Review and Summary

Risk management is an organizational function directed toward preventing loss or controlling liability. It has a dual purpose: first, to eliminate harm to the organization or those with whom it comes in contact; second, to reduce the cost associated with these harmful situations.

The external environment of the hospital is becoming more hostile. This hostility is aggravated by escalating cost, organizational complexity, ultraspecialization, and public expectations. Public accountability is being demanded and, at the same time, susceptibility to liability hazards is increasing.

The dynamics of the hospitals are also changing the *internal* disposition of hospitals. Organizational family life is becoming more complicated and creating multitudinous people problems. The roles of the many individuals and staffs involved in hospital-related activities seem to conflict at times, which adds to confusion within institutions.

In the midst of all these complicated circumstances, endless increases in cost seem to be the rule. One of the significant contributors to these increases is liability insurance premiums. To combat this particular problem, new approaches to insuring against liability claims are being tried. Some of these include captive and self-insurance plans, going bare, and innovative commercial insurance programs. However, a common ingredient being found more and more in all these approaches is a new function called risk management.

Risk management is, by definition, a management program. Therefore, defined management processes must be followed to insure its effectiveness. Though *risk* has a negative connotation and implies the need for avoidance and *management* is considered an active effort to achieve positive results, the term risk management is not paradoxical. It is, instead, a part of a good overall management program.

A helpful exercise to conduct prior to initiating a formal risk management

131

program in a hospital is an inventory of the existing operational activities that will relate to such a program. These activities will form the base on which a program can be developed. These activities or prerequisites fall into five basic categories: preventive, corrective, documentary, educational, and administrative.

Preventive activities generally include those that promote quality service within the hospital. Meaningful patient, public, personnel, and medical staff relations programs are prime examples of preventive activities. Additionally, functions that improve the physical environment and promote safety and security also fit in this category.

Corrective activities include not only remedying existing problem situations that have occurred but also seeking out and solving hidden or potential risk problems. The identification of risks, the use of defined investigative techniques, the instigation of remedial action, and the incorporation of monitoring and audit procedures are classified as corrective.

The *documentation* of all aspects of hospital operations is an important prerequisite to a risk management program. The formal record is crucial, not only from a quality but also from a continuity standpoint. An inventory of recordkeeping is helpful and generally reflective of operational competence.

Education is another organization function that is critical if a risk management program is contemplated. It must perform three related roles: first, provide staff and patient training; second, orient hospital and medical staffs to operational systems and conduct skills training in the various components of the system; third, be responsive to operational needs through continuing education.

Effective *administration* within an institution as complex as a hospital is the final requirement. The existence of an administrative philosophy that is understood and practiced throughout the hospital lends necessary support to any new program. An administration that permeates the organization, is active, uses good judgment, communicates, creates organizational motion, and is based on sound operational principles is an important key to the success of any hospital and its programs.

The establishment of a risk management program within the hospital organizational structure can be accomplished in many ways. Some basic guidelines should be considered. First, a risk management program should be coordinated with and enhance existing activities. Second, risk management should be recognized as basically a staff function. Third, the program should be broad in scope. Fourth, adequate commitment is necessary for the program to succeed. Fifth, risk management should justify its existence from both service and fiscal standpoints.

The administrator of the risk management program is the risk manager. The person carrying this responsibility plays a unique role that requires special skills and talents. The program structured under the risk manager's leadership should incorporate and coordinate existing committee activities related to safety and loss control as well as quality assurance. It is important that an integration of committee functions take place to insure effectiveness and eliminate duplication. Such committees as environmental control and energy conservation, fire safety, employee safety, patient and public safety, disaster, security, infections control, education, and patient care evaluation should be involved in the coordination of effort.

Appropriate policies and procedures should be formulated in conjunction with the risk management program. General policy, standard, personnel, and departmental policies and procedures must be consistent with the purposes and objectives of the program. Many policies and procedures probably already exist and may need only minor adaptation to conform to the program.

Risk management is a team function. The important members of this team include the governing body and administration, risk manager, department heads, employees and other workers, related committees, members of the medical staff, hospital attorney, and risk management consultants (if any). Each of these play important yet different roles in risk management activities. A cooperative and supportive attitude by each will insure maximum program effectiveness.

Although the physical location may vary, the risk management office serves as a central clearinghouse for information as well as the liability control center. It should not be considered as just a receiver of information but, more importantly, as an initiator of appropriate action directed toward prevention and correction.

One of the primary responsibilities of the risk management program is the handling of potential liability problems. The several steps involved in this function include problem identification, screening, review, analysis, resolution, follow-up, and, when necessary, litigation preparation.

The primary tools used in the identification of problems are incident/accident reports. However, other methods are also necessary to insure discovery of problems. Policies and procedures should not only spell out the definition of incidents and accidents but also pinpoint responsibilities involved in their identification. The centralization of related information is desirable and adds to the effectiveness of the liability control system.

The division of problem situations into major and minor classifications is important so that the greatest effort can be devoted to the most serious incidents/accidents. As a part of this process, personal contact with those involved can be crucial to the ultimate outcome. Therefore, certain interpersonal skills and talents need to be fully developed and utilized.

In reviewing, analyzing, and, hopefully, resolving problems, additional techniques and tools may prove helpful, including checklists, summary sheets, and other special purpose forms. In regard to individual problems, several courses of action relative to the hospital's stance on each incident/accident are available. These include (1) accepting no responsibility, (2) accepting limited responsibility, (3) accepting total responsibility, and (4) accepting necessary responsibility. From a general standpoint, problem situations must be reviewed and analyzed to determine trends and patterns.

When litigation becomes inevitable, good preparation, judgment, and strategy are indispensable. Certain administrative principles relating to the litigation process should be followed. However, the need for competence and knowledgeability on the part of the hospital's legal counsel cannot be overemphasized. Remember that the hospital's track record in the courtroom often will have a direct bearing on future exploitation of risk situations.

The justification and feasibility of a formal risk management program within an organization must be determined by the individual institution. Many times a truly accurate determination is complicated by the intangible and subjective characteristics inherent in such staff services as risk management. In spite of its impalpable nature, a risk management program may have even greater potential than other staff services. One reason is the current high cost of liability. Another reason is the fact that so many of the activities involved in the risk management function already exist in most hospitals and only need redirection and coordination.

Some of the factors that have a direct bearing on feasibility and justification include (1) the type of insurance program currently in force, (2) the size and scope of the hospital, (3) risk history and experience, (4) community attitudes, and (5) demographics. An analysis and review of each of these factors will assist in clarifying each hospital's decision in regard to risk management as an organizational function.

The formulation of a budget and the determination of related expenses are initial steps in program evaluation. The relationship of these expenditures to total institutional cost places the program in better perspective from a financial standpoint.

A more significant aspect of the justification/ feasibility evaluation is the *service* provided by a risk management program. The social responsibility of the hospital is a factor that must be considered in program analysis. Risk management offers great potential nonfinancial benefits to a hospital.

Risk management is a program that has application regardless of the type of insurance program in force in a hospital. However, if a hospital chooses to establish a self-insurance plan, it is imperative that a risk management program be initiated concurrently. There are two basic reasons for this requirement. First, risk prevention activities reduce possible harm to all those associated with the hospital, with resultant cost savings. Second, the Medicare Bureau requires that self-insuring hospitals have risk management programs if they wish to have fund contributions treated as allowable cost.

The approach to self-insurance may vary with each hospital. One may select to self-insure only a portion of the institution's risk exposure, whereas another may decide to totally self-insure. When evaluating this decision, it is also important to remember that general and professional liability coverage cannot be easily separated.

There are generally two basic reasons for a hospital to select the self-insurance route. First, such insurance purchased commercially is too costly, and second, malpractice insurance (at any price) may not be available. Also, some authorities suggest that the insurance premium cost must be significantly high before an institution can accept the risk associated with a self-insurance plan.

Several necessary documents must be developed to meet Medicare requirements for an approved self-insurance program. Two of the important ones are the self-insurance plan and the restricted trustee agreement. In addition, annual actuarial studies must be performed to establish appropriate funding levels. The legal aspects of meeting institutional obligations, such as bond agreements and resolutions, must also be taken into consideration when evaluating the implementation of self-insurance within a hospital.

An intriguing psychological impact may result from both self-insurance and risk management programs. Internal as well as external attitudes toward the hospital may be positively affected by such programs if they are conceived, developed, and utilized in the proper mode.

In summary, basic decisions related to hospital operations are the main determinants of long-range institutional success. In this regard, all hospital administrators are desirous of making good decisions that will insure their hospitals the right to enjoy a healthy, progressive, vital existence.

Many of these decisions are difficult, particularly when they involve the initiation or expansion of costly operational activities. Determining priorities for the use of limited resources to satisfy seemingly unlimited demands becomes an agonizing process. What will this new function do for us? Is this activity more important than the others being proposed? Is the timing right for such a program? These are some of the questions that will run through administrators' minds.

Risk management in the hospital setting is an idea whose time has come. Such a program is no longer a luxury; it is now a necessity. The real question is not *whether* to begin, but rather *how* to proceed. This author has attempted to place a practical tool in the hands of governing bodies, administrators, and staffs to assist in efforts to establish and/or refine risk management programs within their hospitals.

Glossary

RISK MANAGEMENT TERMINOLOGY AND RELATED NOMENCLATURE

This glossary includes definitions that relate to risk management in the hospital setting. A glossary such as this cannot provide a short course in such a subject as risk management. Instead, this particular glossary attempts to provide a standard meaning in the context of risk management for those related items that are included. Its object is to enable people to communicate more effectively with each other concerning this timely subject. To a large extent, nontechnical language is used by design in an attempt to increase understanding. It should also be emphasized that these definitions relate to the previous text, which outlines risk management as a hospital function.

Accident: a risk situation or unusual event involving possible harm to employees.[1]

Accident report: form used to document an accident. Must be completed for all accidents.

Actuarial study: determination of funding level for self-insurance trust. Must be performed by a recognized actuary.

Administrative activities: those functions involved in the management and supervision of hospital activities. Should be supportive of the risk management program.

Administrative personnel exchange (APE): a formal program established to provide an exchange of ideas between the frontline employees and top administration in the organization.[2]

Claim: demand made against the hospital or its agents; usually precipitated by an incident or accident occurring within the hospital.

Claims adjustment: settlement of claims resulting from risk situations without litigation; a function usually handled by insurance company, consultant, or claims management committee.

Commercial insurance: conventional purchased insurance plan obtained through a licensed carrier.

Corrective activities: those functions that not only remedy existing problem situations, but also seek out and solve hidden or potential risk problems.

Departmental policy and procedure (DPP): all intradepartmental policies, procedures, and instructions usually recorded in departmental manuals.

Documentary activities: formalization of records and reports relative to hospital operations; crucial from a quality as well as a continuity standpoint.

Education activities: those functions that orient, train, educate, and promote better understanding among all persons working at or served by the hospital.

Employee recognition: activities designed to recognize and reward employees for excellent service; an excellent motivation tool.

General liability: includes risk responsibility not specifically included in other types of liabilities; normally included in conjunction with a professional liability insurance program.

General policy: the policy established by the governing body of an organization based on broad goals and objectives of the institution; serves as a guide for other organizational policies and procedures.

Going bare: without any type of insurance program or plan. An option some hospitals are choosing because of the unavailability and/or high cost of commercial insurance.

Hospital attorney: legal counsel and advisor to the hospital. A member of the risk management team.

Hospital slogan: motto or credo reflecting the hospital purpose, objective, and/or philosophy.

Incident: a risk situation or unusual happening involving patients, visitors, volunteers, and the general public.[3]

Incident report: form used to document an incident. Must be completed for all incidents.

Liability control: see **Risk management.**

Liability control center: central clearinghouse for liability information and coordination center for liability related activities.[4]

Line service: a department or function that usually provides a direct service to the hospital's customers and consumers.

Loss prevention: see **Risk management.**

Malpractice: see **Professional liability.**

Management by objectives: management technique used to promote efficiency and effectiveness of organizational activities; includes the establishment of functional purpose, accomplishments, objectives, and necessary resources.

Medical staff opinion poll: an opinion survey conducted periodically to determine attitudes of physicians on the medical staff relative to hospital operational activities.[5]

Medical staff relations: activities designed to improve physicians' attitudes toward the hospital and involve them in its operations.

Ombudsmen: representatives of the hospital who provide direct liaison with and assistance to patients in addition to regular hospital employees; patient representatives.

Patient relations: activities designed to improve patient attitudes toward the hospital and the quality of service provided by it.

Patient service questionnaire: survey form used to obtain patient evaluation of hospital services. Results should be distributed to those providing such services as well as to the governing body.

Personnel policy and procedure (PPP): all interorganizational policies, procedures, and instructions of a personnel and employment nature usually centralized in an institutional manual.

Personnel relations: activities designed to improve employees' attitudes toward the hospital and their jobs, which hopefully will result in improved patient services.

Policy: basic principles or guidelines that govern and direct an organization's activities and upon which its procedures are founded.

Preventive activities: activities within the hospital that foster technical as well as personal quality care and seek to accomplish an environment free of risk.

Procedure: operational rules, regulations, and methods based on policies established to provide consistency and direction to organizational activities.

Professional liability: malpractice occurring in the hospital; usually results from negligence or poor judgment on the part of a hospital employee or physician.

Public relations: activities designed to improve public attitudes toward the hospital and promote a good hospital image within the community.

Quality assurance: activities designed to improve and maintain quality service and care; performed through a formal program with involvement of multiple organizational components and committees.

Risk: the probability that something undesirable will happen; implies the need for avoidance.

Risk management: the science of the identification, evaluation, and treatment of financial loss.[6] A program that attempts to provide positive avoidance of negative results. Liability control; loss prevention.

Risk management office: the physical location or headquarters of the risk management program; the risk manager's home base.

Risk management team: includes all those working to reduce risk and problem situations within the hospital: governing body and administration, risk manager, hospital department heads, hospital employees, workers and volunteers, the safety and loss control council/committees, members of the medical staff, hospital attorney, and outside consultants.

Risk manager: person managing or directing the risk management program; coordinator of the hospital's loss-control efforts.

Risk retention: the amount of loss due to liability risk that a hospital retains or absorbs; should be limited to an amount that will not impair its financial strength.[7]

Safety: in the purest sense, free from risk or harm; from a practical standpoint, a policy issue that involves the weighing of properly identified risks and benefits.[8]

Safety and loss control council: overall risk management coordinating group. Composed of such committees as environmental control and energy conservation, fire safety, employee safety, patient and public safety, disaster, education, infection control, and others as needed.

Security: protection from harm caused by unlawful activities and the sense of well-being derived therefrom.

Self-insurance: retaining risk of loss or liability within the organization and providing a funding mechanism to cover cost.

Social responsibility: an institution's sensitivity to providing quality and safe service.

Staff service: a department or function generally advisory in nature that supplements and supports line service activities.

Standard policy and procedure (SPP): all interorganizational policies, procedures, and instructions of a nonpersonnel nature, usually centralized in an institutional manual.

Trust: a mechanism to fund a self-insurance program; must be restricted and its funding level actuarially determined to receive maximum reimbursement from federal programs.

Workmen's compensation: payment to employees resulting from job-related injury or illness.

REFERENCES

1. G. Newman, "Basic elements of a Loss Control Program," *Hospital Progress,* November 1974, p. 49.
2. A. Bennett, "Focus on Management Methods," *Hospital Topics,* August 1973, p. 16.
3. Newman, p. 49.
4. *Controlling Hospital Liability: A Systems Approach,* developed and written by the Maryland Hospital Education Institute (Chicago: American Hospital Association, 1976), p. 2.
5. B. Brown, "Staff Opinion Polls," *Hospitals, JAHA,* June 16, 1970, p. 70.

6. T. Dankmyer and J. Groves, "Taking Steps for Safety's Sake," *Hospitals, JAHA,* May 16, 1977, p. 60.
7. A. Clark, "Management Approaches to Basic Risks," *Hospital Progress,* November 1974, p. 43.
8. C. Epting, "Of Mice and Men: Health Risks and Safety Judgments," *Facts and Issues, League of Women Voters,* 1977, p. 1.

Practical Applications Through Case Studies

Possibly the most effective tool to use in demonstrating the practical approach or application of a program is through the use of actual case studies. Appendix A attempts to demonstrate a risk management program in action. The cases described will include a variety of actual situations; of course, the facts and circumstances have been changed somewhat to maintain anonymity. The language used is typical of that found on incident/accident reports and other related forms. No implication is intended that the handling of these situations as presented is the *right* or the *only* way. Instead, the purpose of these cases is to describe methodology and approach that resulted from a functioning risk management program.

CASE 1—A VISITOR FALL

1. Pertinent information from Incident Report:

Name: Code 1978-151-V
Date: 10-9-78
Time: 12:30 P.M.
Age: 66 years
Category: Visitor
Address: 123 Second Street, City
Occupation: Housewife
Exact location of incident: Room 519 (husband's room)
Employee's account of incident: Visitor stated she slipped in water or something wet. She was found lying on floor with left foot twisted at the ankle. She was sent to E.R.
Witness: Husband, the patient
Physician's statement: Fracture, dislocation of left ankle. Admitted to Room 530.

2. Other statements included:

I heard someone call for help and I saw an orderly and other personnel go into room 519. Mrs. S was on the floor on her back and her left ankle was at an abnormal angle. She was in stocking feet (no shoes) and her shoes were near the wall. There was a partially eaten sandwich with two pieces on the floor. A small palm size wet area was near her right shoulder. Mrs. S was complaining of pain in her left ankle. Her ankle was splinted and she was lifted to a stretcher and sent to E.R.

(Registered Nurse)

When I was in the room (519) earlier, I didn't see anything on the floor. The room was in normal condition. Mrs. S offered to finish feeding her husband. I left the room at approximately 11:55 A.M.

(Nursing Assistant)

Other statements similar.

Diagram of the area was prepared indicating location of patient bed, chair, sandwich on floor, small wet area, shoes, and where Mrs. S was lying.

3. Action taken and resolution:

After immediate problem was handled, risk manager was informed and statements and other information gathered.

Surgery was necessary on Mrs. S.

Information was forwarded to the hospital attorney.

Hospital was contacted by family concerning liability insurance to cover the incident.

Emergency care charges were waived per hospital policy. Other costs were covered by patient's insurance.

Incident was reviewed and evaluated by Patient and Public Safety Committee, and judgment was made that the hospital should not accept responsibility for any additional cost as a result of this incident (*accept no responsibility*). It was felt that no negligence on the part of hospital staff existed in this case. The wet area was evidently the result of spillage caused by Mrs. S.

Risk Manager with the Director of Nursing discussed this incident with the family, indicating that the hospital had investigated the incident in detail and as a courtesy was waiving the cost for immediate emergency care per its policy.

Fortunately, in this case the family members understood and agreed with the decision made, were grateful for the waived charges and the attention and attitude of the hospital staff.

CASE 2—LOSS OF DENTURES

1. Pertinent information from Incident Report:

Name: Code 1977-128-P
Date: 8-27-77
Time: 11:30 A.M.
Age: 78 years
Category: Patient
Exact location of incident: Room 548
Employee's account of incident: When patient's belongings were packed to transfer patient to Intensive Care Unit after surgery, dentures were placed in denture cup and placed in admission kit by nursing assistant to carry to ICU. It was left in room. However, ICU personnel states no admission kit was received and a new kit was obtained for the patient.

(Registered Nurse)

2. Other statements included:

We have been unable to locate the dentures and the family expresses concern. I feel the teeth, which were in the admission kit along with house slippers, were discarded.

(ICU Nurse)

Remember seeing admissions kit in 548. It did not have a denture cup or slippers in it. The bath basin containing pitchers, soap dish, and emesis basin was discarded.

(Housekeeping Supervisor)

From critical incident investigation form: Mr. B (son) came by the nursing office to express concern related to his mother's dentures, which were lost. He stated that the doctor has indicated that his mother was in critical condition and could not consider denture replacement at this time. Therefore, he planned to send us a copy of the bill of the original teeth. I advised him that this would be reviewed and we would be back in touch with him. Son praised care his mother had received during her stay.

(Director of Nursing)

3. Other information:

Patient expired within one week.

4. Action taken and resolution:

Risk Manager notified of incident and attempts were made to recover the dentures through the Housekeeping Department with no success.

During the course of review and analysis, patient expired. Therefore, there was no need for the dentures.

Reviewed by the Patient and Public Safety Committee, which recommended that the hospital accept no responsibility unless pressed by the family (*accept necessary responsibility*). Additionally, the committee asked that the procedure used in the handling of dentures be reviewed by Nursing Service. As a result, the procedure was improved and such incidents reduced.

The hospital ultimately paid the estate $650, which was the original cost of the dentures. A general release from liability was obtained when the settlement was made.

CASE 3—MEDICATION ERROR

1. Pertinent information from Incident Report:

Name: Code 1978-042-P
Date: 3-6-78
Time: 10:30 A.M.
Age: 56 years
Category: Patient
Exact location of incident: Room 616
Cause of hospitalization: lymphoma
Employee account of incident: Administered IV medication to Mr. C in error; he was the wrong patient.

<u>(Registered Nurse, IV team)</u>

2. From Medication and Treatment Errors and Omission form:

I entered patient's room, addressing him verbally as Mr. K; I identified myself and told him why I was here. I asked him if his doctor had discussed his treatment with him and received a positive response. I explained again what I was going to do; called the patient "Mr. K" during the whole conversation. I then completed the venipuncture, gave the medicine, and charted on the chart, which was laying out for me on the desk.

When the night nurse came on duty, Mr. K and his wife said he had not received his medication. She inquired with other personnel and was able to ascertain that Mr. C had been the recipient since he had a venipuncture. She had called me when Mr. K had first reported his omission. When she found out who had gotten the drug, she notified Mr. C's doctor and called Mr. K's doctor.

3. Other information:

Mr. C was in room 616 and Mr. K was in room 618.

The addressograph imprint on Mr. K's order looked like room 616 and the nurse, because of this, had gone to the wrong room.

The nurse did not check the patient's armband, which is part of the procedure.

3. Action taken and resolution:

Risk Manager with the Nursing Supervisor reviewed the incident with the doctors involved. Both felt no harm would result from error; however, Mr. C's doctor felt he should remain in the hospital for two extra days for observation.

Doctor and Nursing Supervisor discussed the error with the patient and his wife, and they accepted the explanation and were not upset. However, they did not feel that they should pay the hospital bill for the extra days.

Reviewed by the Patient and Public Safety Committee, which recommended discounting the extra cost resulting from the extended stay (*accept limited responsibility*).

The hospital accepted the recommendation of the committee and discounted two days of hospital stay.

The nurse received counseling in regard to procedure and consequence of an error such as this.

CASE 4—PRODUCT LIABILITY

1. Pertinent information from Incident Report:

Name: Code 1976-012-P
Date: 1-20-76
Time: 3:00 P.M.
Age: 33 years
Category: Patient
Cause of hospitalization: urethral stones
Equipment involved: cysto stone dislodger
Employee's account of incident: While attempting stone extraction, stone basket was dislodged.

(O.R. Nurse)

Doctor is talking with patient's family about the incident and will surgically remove wires. I am attempting to contact the manufacturer's representative.

(O.R. Supervisor)

Physician's account of incident: After stone basket was inserted and opened without difficulty, when the basket was withdrawn, the basket wires were gone. No undue resistance or pressure was applied to the faulty basket.

(Surgeon)

2. Other information:

Within a week, after surgery was performed to remove wires with no complications, letter was received from patient's attorney requesting the faulty instrument be retained. This was being done in expectation of the request.

Manufacturer of the instrument was foreign. Therefore, attempts failed to contact. Sales representative who no longer called on the hospital was notified, but disclaimed any responsibility.

3. Action taken and resolution:

Risk Manager with the doctor and Operating Room Supervisor reviewed the incident. It was referred to the Patient and Public Safety Committee.

Doctor explained the incident in detail to the patient and family, explaining the malfunction of the equipment.

Because the repercussions to the patient were fortunately minor (discomfort, extended hospital stay, slight delay in returning to work), a fairly positive attitude was exhibited.

The Patient and Public Safety Committee recommended that added cost to the patient's hospital bill be discounted and that, if the patient requested, a small payment for lost work time be paid (*accept necessary responsibility*). The Committee also recommended that the hospital attorney, if determined feasible, should begin legal action against the manufacturer and sales representative in regard to this situation. If further settlement was necessary, it was recommended that the surgeon be requested to assist in these expenses.

Additionally, the Committee recommended a purchasing policy be developed relative to the acquisition of instruments, equipment, and supplies that are manufactured and/or sold to the hospital from foreign organizations or those unfamiliar to the institution.

CASE 5—SITUATION WITH SERIOUS CONSEQUENCES

1. Pertinent information from Incident Report:

Name: Code 1978-061-P
Date: 4-12-78
Time: 10:35 A.M.
Age: 2 years
Category: Patient (E.R.)
Reason for presence in hospital: possible fracture
Employee account of incident: Camera magazine in room #8 after being released, fell and bounced off the table and landed on child's head. Child was lying on the table and I was holding her still with one hand (trying to help get films run so we could check them and let the patient go) when released magazine fell and bounced on the table, then hit the child's head resulting in fracture of right side of the skull.

(Radiologic Technologist)

I came out from behind the control booth and met Dr. A on his way out of the room. We were comparing the size and shape of an identity card with computer card. Miss B (other technician) was left in the room with the child. She was attempting to remove the film holder with her left hand while holding the child on the table with her right hand. Dr. A and I were at the doorway when I decided to go back to the table to assist Miss B. I turned and started back to the table when I noticed the film holder lying on what appeared to be the child's right shoulder. I ran to the front of the table to see what had happened. When I reached the head of the x-ray table, I noticed a small red mark on the right side of the child's skull.

(Another Technologist)

Statement of physician: When I heard the noise of the magazine hitting the table, I rushed back into the room and took the child who was crying but who stopped shortly. Examination revealed a small bruise on right temporal area. . . . Dr. H (child's pediatrician) was called. X-ray indicated skull fracture. Dr. H and I talked immediately with the child's parents and Dr. S (neurosurgeon) was called.

(Radiologist)

2. Other information:

The neurosurgeon's examination determined the need for corrective surgery. The extent of damage could not be determined.

3. Action taken and resolution:

The Risk Manager, after being notified of the incident, immediately contacted the administrator on call for the weekend. They, with the physicians involved, met to review the case. It was decided that the physician involved would continue in a liaison role with the family.

Corrective surgery was performed the next morning and results appeared good.

Following the resolution of the immediate problem, the Patient and Public Safety Committee held a special called meeting to review this incident. It was the recommendation of the committee that a top hospital official meet with the family and that all medical and related cost be paid by the hospital and a course of *necessary responsibility* be followed.

Of greatest concern to the family was any permanent damage that might result from the incident, yet initially, be undeterminable. The administrator agreed with this concern and pledged support in obtaining available diagnostic services to alleviate this apprehension. During the following eighteen months, specialty services were provided at the hospital's expense and no permanent problems were determined.

Approximately two years after the incident, the hospital was contacted by an attorney for the family seeking a financial settlement. After negotiation, the hospital claims management committee approved a small settlement of the case at which time a release from liability was signed by the family.

CASE 6—EMPLOYEE ACCIDENT

1. Pertinent information:

No Accident Report was completed initially.

Employee when leaving the hospital building after clocking out at approximately 11:15 P.M. fell on iced area outside the exit. Two other employees witnessed the accident; however, there was no apparent injury so they all left without reporting the mishap.

Approximately a week later the employee who fell called her supervisor and indicated that her back was "hurting" her and requested a few days off under workmen's compensation.

Supervisor with consultation granted the time off but indicated that the workmen's compensation coverage would have to be determined after investigating the accident.

2. Action taken and resolution:

Risk manager requested accident report be completed by the employee's supervisor and statements be obtained from witnesses of the accident.

Employee was told that failure to immediately report the accident per hospital policy could jeopardize a claim under the hospital's workmen's compensation program.

Risk manager interviewed the injured employee in depth about the accident. In the course of the interview the employee indicated that she fell again approximately a week later at home and reinjured her back. A statement including this additional information was prepared and signed by the employee.

Employee was again told that failure to immediately report the accident violated hospital policy.

Employee Safety Committee reviewed the accident and recommended (a) a workmen's compensation claim not be made since the additional fall which occurred at home made it impossible to distinguish whether the fall at the hospital resulted in injury, (b) that the employee be granted sick leave for days missed if she was due any under the hospital's accrual system.

Employee was informed by the risk manager and accepted the hospital's decision.

New emphasis was given through organizational channels to the policy of immediate reporting of incidents and accidents.

CASE 7—MEDIA PROBLEM

1. Brief description of the problem:

The hospital's Public Relations Director received a telephone call from a local television news personality who specialized in investigative reporting on consumer abuse. This reporter indicated that he had been contacted and told of an incident which occurred in the hospital resulting in a serious injury to a patient. He wanted to know the condition of the patient to include in a report on the hospital's negligence which was being taped for the evening news. He also stated that he would be happy for a hospital representative to be interviewed to explain the institution's position. The Public Relations Director initially invoked the hospital's policy relative to the confidentiality of medical records and patient privacy. However, to preserve a good relationship which the hospital had enjoyed with this T.V. station, she indicated that she would call back after checking into the situation.

The Administrator was contacted immediately who, in turn, asked the Risk Manager to review the incident which had occurred several days earlier. After a briefing relative to the incident, the hospital attorney was also consulted. It was determined that the reporter's facts were fairly accurate but, at the same time, his interpretation was somewhat biased. The patient was doing well and suffered no apparent ill effects from the incident.

The choices seemed to be: (a) refuse to talk with the reporter and take a chance on the news report being objective and nondamaging, or (b) talk with the reporter and run the risk of publicly reviewing a hospital incident. Of course, the hospital's position was that such situations should never be resolved on a television news program. It was also felt that the institution's reputation and image could suffer immeasurable damage irrespective of the objectivity and accuracy of the report.

2. Action taken and resolution:

After reviewing the situation with members of the risk management team, it was determined that the Administrator with the Risk Manager would talk with the reporter. However, certain stipulations would be made. These included (a) the conversation would not be taped, (b) the content of the conversation would be "off the record" and not included in the report, and (c) if the reporter continued the report after receiving the hospital's explanation, he would do so without the hospital's participation. The reporter agreed to all of these provisions.

The basic facts of the incident were reviewed (which were already known to him). Emphasis was given to the following points: (a) the incident was the result of human error and the persons involved had years of experience with no record of negligence, (b) possible litigation could occur from a situation such as this and inappropriate publicity could improperly influence any such action, (c) the hospital intended to be fair with those involved in the incident and accept appropriate responsibility, and (d) the hospital was sympathetic to consumer abuse reporting, however, this incident had happened only a few days before and adequate time had not been given to satisfactorily resolve the incident with the patient and family.

The reporter listened thoughtfully to the entire explanation and left after stating that he also intended to be "fair." No report was ever made on television of the incident.

Composition of Safety and Loss Control Council

The following is an example of the way in which a Safety and Loss Control Council might be organized.

*Chairperson—Director of safety, security, and loss prevention (risk manager) ex-officio member of all committees
Secretary—appointment member
*Advisor—hospital attorney
*Medical staff representative(s)

Committees(within the Council)

1. Environment Control and Energy Conservation
   *Director of housekeeping—chairperson
   *Maintenance—supervisory
   Housekeeping—supervisory
   Central supply—nonsupervisory
   Others as needed

2. Fire Safety
   *Director of engineering—chairperson
   *Nursing service—nonsupervisory
   Laundry—supervisory
   Laboratory—nonsupervisory
   Others as needed

3. Employee Safety
   *Director of Personnel—chairperson
   *Employee health nurse
   Infections control—supervisory
   Nursing service—nonsupervisory

*Permanent member.

Food service—nonsupervisory
*Medical staff—employee health
Others as needed

4. Patient and Public Safety
   *Assistant administrator, patient services—chairperson
   *Patient accounts—supervisory
   Nursing service—nonsupervisory
   Administration—nonsupervisory
   *Medical staff—patient care
   Others as needed

5. Disaster
   *Nursing supervisor—chairperson
   Emergency services—nonsupervisory
   Admissions—nonsupervisory
   Surgical suite—nonsupervisory
   *Medical staff—emergency service and/or medical disaster committee
   Others as needed

6. Education
   *Director of educational services—chairperson
   *Public affairs—supervisory
   Educational services—nonsupervisory
   Respiratory therapy—nonsupervisory
   *Medical staff—medical education
   Others as needed

7. Security
   *Security officer—chairperson
   *Nursing service—supervisory
   Security—nonsupervisory
   Pharmacy—nonsupervisory
   Others as needed

8. Infections Control
   *Pathologist—chairperson
   *Infections control nurse
   *Director of housekeeping
   *Central service—supervisory
   Nursing service—nonsupervisory
   Surgery—nonsupervisory
   Others as needed

(Infections Control Committee may be part of the quality assurance program, provided it is multidisciplined and hospital-wide in composition to meet JCAH standards.)

9. Others (as needed)

In addition to officers, council meetings should be attended by the chairperson and all permanent members from each committee. Others may be included as needed.

Example of a Self-Insurance Plan

Whereas, for the past several years the Hospital Governing Body (herein referred to as "Governing Body") of _____ Hospital has purchased liability insurance which included hospital professional and general liability coverage; and

Whereas, such policy included professional liability and general liability coverage for the defense and payment of loss as specified in such liability insurance policy; and

Whereas, premiums quoted for insurance, equivalent to that previously provided, were excessive and not justified hospital experience in claim losses and expenses; and

Whereas, the Governing Body has been unable to secure adequate insurance at fair and reasonable premium rates; and

Whereas, it has been determined that the most reasonable and prudent course for the Governing Body is to provide self-insurance,

Now, therefore, the Governing Body does hereby establish this Self-Insurance Plan (hereinafter referred to as "Plan"), as follows:

1. Coverage:

Effective _____, the Governing Body operates as a self-insured. Pursuant to the provisions of this Plan, and subject to the terms and conditions hereof, coverage shall include:

a. Payment of sums which the Governing Body shall become legally obligated to pay as damages resulting from the course of the Governing Body's operations, but only to the extent such legal obligations are not otherwise covered by insurance.

b. Payment of those sums which are the legal obligation of the following when incurred while acting for or on behalf of the Governing Body: employees, officers, students, and trainees assigned to the Governing

Body, authorized volunteer workers, members of medical committees, and trustees. Such coverage does not include bodily injury to any employee arising out of and in the course of his employment of the Governing Body.

c. The total limit of payments under this Plan for all personnel described in subparagraph (b.) above is _____ per occurrence and _____ aggregate during the period of beginning fiscal year through ending fiscal year of each consecutive year while this Plan is in effect. There is excluded from coverage in said subparagraph (b.) any claim arising out of any dishonest, fraudulent or criminal act and claims for damage or injury willfully inflicted.

d. In addition to the payments under subparagraph (b.) as provided for herein, the Governing Body shall have the right and duty to defend any suit as to which such coverage is applicable and make such investigations and settlement of any claim or suit as it deems desirable. Coverage under this Plan includes the expenses involved in any such defense and settlement including, but not limited to, attorney's fees, investigation costs, interest on judgments, appeal costs, etc. Payment shall not be required of any judgment or settlement or for defense of any suit after the total limit of payment specified in subparagraph (c.) has been exhausted by payments of judgments and settlements.

2. Funding:

This Plan shall be funded (Fund) in an amount to be determined by the Governing Body in accordance with an independent actuarial determination. Each year thereafter, there shall be deposited in said Fund an amount to be determined by the Governing Body in accordance with independent actuarial determinations. The total amount of the Fund to be ultimately established and maintained shall take into consideration the amount, if any, of excess coverage obtained through an insurance policy or policies.

3. Supervision of Fund:

The Fund herein created shall be administered and invested under the supervision of a trustee determined by the Governing Authority consistent with state and federal requirements.

4. Administration of the Plan:

The general administration of the Plan shall be as provided for by the Administrator of _____ Hospital. Without limiting the foregoing, it is directed that procedures shall be established for, among other things, the following:

  a. The continued filing of incident reports and their review through the risk management program. Policies, procedures and methods shall also be established for the initiation of further investigation of and follow-up on all incident reports by appropriate reviewing parties;
  b. The review of all claims and settlement recommendations by designated hospital staff members, committees, and hospital counsel;
  c. The design and implementation of a safety and loss prevention program under a risk manager. Outside services may be contracted for to assist with the design, implementation, monitoring and evaluation of such program.

5. Purposes for which Plan may be used:

Withdrawals from this Plan from funds held by the Trustee must be for malpractice and comprehensive general liability losses of the hospital only but shall include the following expenses:

  a. Expenses of establishing this Self-Insurance Plan;
  b. Expenses for administering the Claims Management Program;
  c. Expenses involved in maintenance of the fund of the Trustee;
  d. Legal expenses;
  e. Excess insurance coverage (if purchased by Governing Body);
  f. Applicable risk management expenses.

The foregoing expenses are payable provided such expenses are related to this Plan. All other expenses will not be considered cost attributable to this Plan but shall be included in Governing Body administration and general cost in the year incurred. Any rebates, dividends, or like amounts flowing to the hospital from this Plan shall be used to reduce allowable cost.

Payments under this Plan, and authorizations to the Governing Body for such payments shall be by the unanimous concurrence of the Claims Management Committee consisting of:

  a. Chairman of the Governing Body
  b. Hospital administrator
  c. Hospital Attorney
  d. Risk Manager (advisory without vote)

All of the signatures of the members of the Claims Management Committee shall be continuously on file with the Trustee. The signatures of any two (2) members of the Claims Management Committee shall be required by the Trustee for withdrawal from the fund.

6. Conditions:

Any Party becoming aware of any possible injury or loss or damage to which the coverage under this Plan may apply, shall give written notice containing particulars sufficient to identify the Party and include reasonably obtainable information with respect to the time, place and circumstances thereof, and the names and addresses of the injured and of available witnesses. Such notice shall be given by or for the Party to the office of the Administrator, his designate or the Risk Manager as soon as practicable. As used herein Party refers to any individual included in the coverage described in Paragraph I and the subparagraphs thereof.

If claim is made or suit is brought against a Party, such Party shall immediately forward to the Governing Body every demand, notice, summons or other process received by him or his representative.

All interested Parties shall cooperate with the Governing Body and, upon Authority's request, assist in making settlements, in the conduct of suits and in enforcing any right of contribution or indemnity against any person or organization who may be liable to Parties at interest because of injury or damage with respect to which coverage under this Plan applies; and Parties at interest shall attend hearings, trials and assist in securing and giving evidence and obtaining the attendance of witnesses. Parties at interest shall not, except at their own cost, voluntarily offer or voluntarily make any payment, assume any obligation or incur any expense other than first aid to others at the time of accident.

No action shall lie against the Authority unless, as a condition precedent thereto, there shall have been full compliance with all the terms and conditions of this Plan, nor until the amount of the Party's obligation to pay shall have been finally determined either by judgment against the Party after actual trial or by written agreement of the Party, the claimant and the Governing Body.

Any person or organization or the legal representative thereof who has secured such judgment or written agreement shall thereafter be entitled to recover under this Plan to the extent stated herein. No person or organization shall have any right under this Plan to join the Governing Body as a party to any action against a Party at interest to determine such Party's liability, nor shall the Authority be impleaded by such Party or his legal representative. Bankruptcy or insolvency of a Party or such Party's estate shall not relieve the Governing Body of any of its obligations hereunder.

In the event of any payment under this Plan, the Governing Body shall be subrogated to all of the Party's rights of recovery therefore against person or organization and the Party shall execute and deliver instruments and papers and do whatever else is necessary to secure such rights. The Party at interest shall do nothing after loss to prejudice such rights.

The interest hereunder of any Party is not assignable. If the Party shall die or be adjudged incompetent, then, as to such Party, coverage under this Plan shall thereupon terminate, but shall extend to the Party's legal representative as the Party with respect to liability previously incurred and covered by this Plan.

Notice of knowledge possessed by employees of the Governing Body, or others, shall not effect a waiver or change in any part of this Plan or stop the Governing Body from asserting any right under the terms of this Plan, nor shall the terms of this Plan be waived or changed, except by the Governing Body's authorized written amendment.

In witness thereof, the Governing Body has caused this Plan to be signed by its Chairman and Secretary and any amendment or termination thereof shall be in writing and similarly signed.

HOSPITAL GOVERNING BODY

_____

Chairman

_____

Secretary

Source: Adapted from the Self-Insurance Plan of Kennestone Hospital, Marietta, Georgia, 1978.

Example of a Trustee Agreement

For the purposes as are hereinafter set forth the Hospital Governing Body of _____ Hospital, hereinafter referred to as "Governing Body," does hereby transfer, deliver, assign and convey to _____(bank or other trustee agent)_____, hereinafter referred to as "Trustee," as Trustee, the property shown on the schedule hereto attached, designated Schedule "A" (funding amounts) and made a part hereof, in trust for the uses and purposes hereinafter set out.

Item I

After the execution of this trust, Governing Body shall have no right, title, or interest in, or power, privilege or incident of ownership in regard to money and/or property in this trust and shall have no right to alter, amend, revoke or terminate this trust or any provision thereof, except as hereinafter provided.

Item II

This trust shall constitute a Self-Insurance Fund, hereinafter referred to as "Fund," established by the Governing Body, with the Trustee having legal title thereto and responsible for its proper administration and control. Investment of the proceeds of this trust shall be made by the Trustee only in such investments as are approved under the Laws of the State of _____ as hereinafter provided; notwithstanding any other provision herein, no loan shall be made to the hospital from the proceeds of this trust.

Item III

The Governing Body shall have the right at any time to add to this trust by depositing additional money with the Trustee hereunder and all such money so deposited shall be held, invested and disbursed by the Trustee in all respects as if it had been a part of the funds originally deposited hereunder, unless the instrument by which such funds are deposited otherwise provides.

Item IV

All income earned by the Trustee from funds deposited in this trust shall be added to and become a part of the corpus of this trust and reinvested by the Trustee as herein provided. Except, that if such Fund, with income earned thereon, shall in the opinion of the actuary, to make said Fund self-perpetuating, then such amount of income annually as shall be determined by the report of the actuary, may be paid over to Governing Body to defray other cost of operation of _____ Hospital.

Item V

Payments by the Trustee, as withdrawals from the trust and income earned thereon, shall be only for malpractice and comprehensive general liability of _____ Hospital, and those expenses related thereto as are set forth in the Governing Body Self-Insurance Plan. Such withdrawals shall be upon written certification by any two (2) members of the Claims Management Committee consisting of:

a. Chairman of the Governing Body
b. Hospital Administrator
c. Hospital Attorney
d. Risk Manager (advisory without vote)

All of the authorized signatures of said Claims Management Committee shall be continuously on file with the Trustee. In the event of the unavoidable absence of one or more of the aforesaid members of the Claims Management Committee, the Governing Body shall be authorized to designate person or persons to temporarily act in substitute capacity as members of the Claims Management Committee.

Item VI

The Trustee shall furnish to Governing Body a financial statement not later than sixty (60) days after the end of each annual insurance reporting period which shall end as of June 30 of each fiscal year. This financial statement must show the balance in the Fund at the beginning of the period, current period contributions, and amount and nature of final payments, including a separate account for claims management, legal expenses, claims paid, other expenses, if any, paid, and the balance in the trust. This annual report and the records of the Trustee shall be available for review and audit; however, the Trustee shall not be required to file annual or other returns to any court, or give bond.

Item VII

An independent actuary, selected by the Governing Body, which actuarial firm shall have actuarial personnel experienced in the field of medical malpractice and general liability insurance, shall prepare an annual certified statement which shall be available for review and filing with appropriate designated offices. The actuary shall determine the amount necessary to be paid into this Self-Insurance Fund. The Fund shall include reserves for losses based on accepted actuarial techniques customarily employed by the casualty insurance industry and expenses related to the self-insurance fund. The actuary shall also provide for an estimate of the amounts to be in excess of that which is reasonably needed to support anticipated disbursements from the Fund.

At such time as the actuary shall certify that all liabilities existent against this Trust have been paid, and the actuary further certified that all claims by actuarial computation have been paid, then upon application by the Governing Body, this Trust may be terminated and all funds remaining in this Trust shall be paid over to the Governing Body to defray other cost of operation of the hospital.

Item VIII

The Trustee shall receive the following compensation: Annual Charges:

First $500,000 market value of assets—$\frac{1}{2}$ of 1% of market value as determined on last portfolio review date; next $500,000.00 market value of assets—$\frac{4}{10}$ of 1%; all over one million dollars ($1,000,000.00)—$\frac{1}{4}$ of 1%; minimum annual charge $500.00.

Item IX

In the management, care and disposition of this trust, the Trustee shall have the power to do all things and to execute such instruments as may be deemed necessary or proper, including the following powers, all of which may be exercised without order of or report to any court:

1. No security or investment shall be eligible for acquisition unless it is interest bearing or interest accruing or dividend or income paying, is not then in default in any respect, and the Trustee is entitled to receive for its account and benefit the interest or income accruing thereon.
2. The Trustee shall not make any investment unless the same is

authorized or approved by the Trustee's Board of Directors or by a committee authorized by such board and charged with the supervision or making of such investment. The minutes of any such committee shall be recorded and regular reports of such committee shall be submitted to the Board of Directors of the Trustee.

3. The Trustee may have as assets, cash or deposits in checking or savings accounts, under certificates of deposit, or in any form in banks and trust companies which have qualified for the insurance protection afforded by the Federal Deposit Insurance Corporation.

4. To the extent that such an investment or account is insured by the Federal Deposit Savings and Loan Insurance Corporation, the Trustee may invest in shares of savings and loan associations or building and loan associations.

5. The Trustee may invest in the securities of any open-end management type investment company or investment trust registered with the Federal Securities and Exchange Commission under the Investment Act of 1940, as from time to time amended, if such investment company or trust has been organized for not less than ten (10) years or has assets of not less than twenty-five million dollars ($25,000,000.00) at the date of investment by the Trustee.

6. The Trustee may invest in obligations issued, assumed, or guaranteed by the International Bank for Reconstruction and Development.

7. The Trustee may invest in bonds, notes, warrants and other evidences of indebtedness which are the direct obligation of the Government of the United States of America or for which the full faith and credit of the Government of the United States of America is pledged for the payment of principal and interest.

8. The Trustee may invest in loans guaranteed as to principal and interest by the Government of the United States, or by any agency or instrumentality of the Government of the United States of America, to the extent of such guaranty.

9. The Trustee may invest in bonds, notes, warrants and other securities not in default which are the direct obligations of any State of the United States or of the District of Columbia, or of the Government of Canada or any province thereof, or for which the full faith and credit of such state, district, government, or province has been pledged for the payment of principal and interest.

10. The Trustee may invest in the obligation of any county, any incorporated city, town, or village, any school district, water district, sewer district, road district, or any other political subdivision in or public authority of any state, territory, or insular provision of the United States, or the District of Columbia, or of the Canadian cities having a

population of over 25,000 according to the most recent official census, which has not defaulted for a period of 120 days in the payment of interest upon, or for a period of more than one (1) year in the payment of principal of, any of its bonds, notes, warrants, certificates of indebtedness, securities, or any other interest-bearing obligation during the five (5) years immediately preceding the acquisition of the investment.

11. The Trustee may invest in the bonds, notes, certificates of indebtedness, warrants or other evidence of indebtedness which are valid obligations issued, assumed or guaranteed by the United States of America or any State thereof, or by any county, municipal corporation, district, or political subdivision, or civil division of public instrumentality of any such government or unit thereof, if by statute or other legal requirements such obligations are payable as to both principal and interest from revenues or earnings from the whole or part of any utility supplying water, gas, sewage disposal facility or electricity or any other public service, including but not limited to toll roads and toll bridges, and in revenue bonds issued by any political subdivision, authority, unit, or other corporate body created by the United States Government or the government of any State, for the purpose of aiding in or promoting the industrial development of such State or political subdivision.

12. The Trustee may invest in bonds, debentures, or other securities issued or insured or guaranteed by any agency, authority, unit or corporate body created by the Government of the United States of America whether or not such obligations are guaranteed by the United States.

13. The Trustee may invest in the bonds, debentures or other securities of public housing authorities, issued under the provisions of the Act of Congress entitled the "Housing Act of 1949" and approved July, 1949; the Municipal Commission Act or the "Rural Housing Commission Act," and any additional amendments, or issued by any other public housing authority or agency in the United States, if such bonds, debentures, or other securities are secured by a pledge of annual contributions to be paid by the United States or by any agency thereof.

14. The Trustee may invest in bonds, debentures, notes and other evidences of indebtedness issued, assumed or guaranteed by any solvent institution existing under the laws of the United States of America or of Canada, or any state or province thereof, which are not in default as to principal or interest and which are secured by collateral worth at least fifty percent (50%) more than the par value of the entire

issue of such obligations, but only if not more than one-third (⅓) of the total value of such required collateral consists of common stocks.

15. The Trustee may invest in equipment trust obligations or certificates adequately secured and evidencing an interest in transportation equipment, wholly or in part within the United States of America, and the right to receive determined portions of rental, purchase, or other fixed obligatory payments for the use of such transportation equipment.

Item X

Notwithstanding any other provision of this Trust, to the extent that this Trust shall fail to meet the Medicare regulations and requirements, then to the extent necessary to comply with federal and state reimbursement program regulations and requirements, this Trust shall be amendable or terminable.

Item XI

The Trustee hereby accepts the trust herein created and agrees to and with the Governing Body in consideration thereof that it will execute the same as herein provided with all due fidelity and that it will account for all monies received and disbursed by it hereunder to Governing Body as herein provided.

It is agreed that the Trustee may resign such Trusteeship on ninety (90) days written notice to Governing Body and, upon properly accounting for all monies received and disbursed by it, be discharged from any and all further liability hereunder.

It is further agreed that Governing Body may upon the giving of ninety (90) days written notice remove said Trust from the Trustee to another successor Trustee of Governing Body's choice.

Item XII

In the event ____ (Trustee) ____ hereafter merges or consolidates with any other bank or trust company, the corporation created by such merger or consolidation shall thereafter act as Trustee hereunder and shall be subject to all the terms and conditions set forth herein.

In witness whereof, the parties hereto have caused this instrument to be signed by its authorized officers, and the corporate seal of each affixed hereto, all on the _____ day of _____, 1978.

THE HOSPITAL'S GOVERNING BODY

BY_____
Chairman

ATTEST_____
Secretary

(SEAL)

Signed, sealed and
delivered in the
presence of:

_____
Witness

_____
Notary Public

_____
Bank or Trustee Agent

BY:_____
Trust Officer

(SEAL)

Signed, sealed and
delivered in the
presence of:

_____
Witness

_____
Notary Public

Source: Adapted from the Trust Agreement of the Self-Insurance Plan of Kennestone Hospital, Marietta, Georgia, 1978.

Selected Bibliography

American Hospital Association. *Risk Management Demonstration Projects.* Chicago: AHA, Tape No. 4565, 1977.

———— *The Incident: Implementing a Hospitalwide Risk Management Program.* Chicago: AHA, 1977.

Cleverley, William O., ed. *Topics in Health Care Financing: Cost Containment Part II.* Germantown, Md.: Aspen Systems Corporation, vol. 3, no. 4, 1977.

Federation of American Hospitals, Inc. *Risk Management Manual: A Guide to Safety, Loss Control, and Malpractice Prevention for Hospitals.* Little Rock, Ark.: FAH, 1977.

Maryland Hospital Education Institute. *Controlling Hospital Liability: A Systems Approach.* Chicago: American Hospital Association, 1976.

Mehr, Robert I., and Hedges, Bob A. *Risk Management: Concepts and Applications.* Homewood, Ill.: Richard D. Irwin, Inc., 1974.

Morse, George P., and Morse, Robert F., II. *Protecting the Health Care Facility: A System of Loss Prevention Management Effective for All Industry.* Baltimore: Williams and Wilkins Company, 1974.

National Safety Council and American Hospital Association. *Safety Guide for Health Care Institutions.* Chicago: NSC/AHA, 1972.

Wood, Jack C., ed. *Topics in Health Care Financing: Risk Management.* Germantown, Md.: Aspen Systems Corporation, vol. 1, no. 4, 1975.

Index

philosophy, 117
policy and procedure development, 61, 62
prerequisites, 9
quality assurance, 9, 119
Safety and Loss Control Council, 56, 57
self-insurance, 124
staff service, 50, 113, 120
structuring, 55
Program, Safety, vi
development, 25, 26
inspection followup memorandum, 33
physical environment, 21
risk manager, 53
Program, Security
development, 25, 26
risk manager, 53
Program, Volunteer
community relations, 13
team approach management, 64
Psychology
self-insurance, 127
impact, 135
Public Relations
community, 13, 14
definition, 139
hospitals, 11
Kindness card, 18
news media, 13

Q

Quality Assurance, xi, 36–38
activities, 139
American Hospital Association Manual, 58
committees, 58, 59, 67
education, 34, 35
improvement, 2
JCAH audits, 34
patient service questionnaire, 12
risk management program, 9, 119
risk manager function, 54
Questionnaire
patient service, 12, 15, 37, 139

R

Recognition
education, 17, 37
Recordkeeping
budget formulation, 111
documentation inventory, 34, 35
incident and accident reports, 89
liability problem handling, 104
See also Documentation
Regulations, vi
physical environment, 21
risk manager, 53
safety, 63
See also Law
Release
further liability, 95
risk manager directed, 54
Remedial Action. See Correction
Reports
accident, 84, 137
centralization, 89, 90
incident, 82, 83, 138
monthly summary, 95, 98, 99
standard policy and procedure, 85–87
inventory, 34, 35
liability problems, 79
trends, 95
management by objectives, 119
occupational injury, 87, 88
office of risk management, 73
problem identification, 81, 133
risk manager, 53
safety and loss control inspection, 28
screening, 90
Responsibility
acceptance, 134
accident reporting, 88
liability problems
limited accepted, 92, 95
necessary accepted, 95
none accepted, 92
total accepted, 95
risk manager, 51-53
social, 114, 134, 140

About the Author

Bernard L. Brown, Jr., FACHA, has been administrator of the 450-bed, ultramodern Kennestone Hospital, Marietta, Georgia, since 1971. After receiving a masters degree in health care administration from George Washington University, Washington, D.C., he held other administrative positions at the University of Alabama Hospitals and Clinics, Birmingham; Memorial Hospital, Gulfport, Mississippi; North Carolina Memorial Hospital, Chapel Hill; and University Hospital, Augusta, Georgia.

He has served in numerous local, state, regional, and national agencies and organizations related to the profession of hospital administration and the health care field. His articles have been published in some of the nation's top professional publications on such subjects as *contract services, personnel relations, medical staff opinions, volunteer orientation, disaster planning, administrative staff organization,* and other related subjects.

Under Mr. Brown's leadership, Kennestone Hospital has won state and national acclaim for its efforts in the area of cost containment (receiving the state PACER award in 1977 and national HFMA Cost Containment award in 1978). It was one of the first hospitals in the state of Georgia and in the southeastern area of the United States to implement a formal self-insurance plan and organize a risk management department, among other innovative and progressive programs.